THE
FAT
ATTACK
PLAN

Books by Annette B. Natow and Jo-Ann Heslin

The Cholesterol Counter
The Fat Attack Plan
The Fat Counter
Megadoses
No-Nonsense Nutrition for Kids
The Pocket Encyclopedia of Nutrition

Published by POCKET BOOKS

THE
FAT
ATTACK
PLAN

ANNETTE B. NATOW, PH.D., R.D.
and JO-ANN HESLIN, M.A., R.D.

POCKET BOOKS
New York   London   Toronto   Sydney   Tokyo   Singapore

POCKET BOOKS, a division of Simon & Schuster Inc.
1230 Avenue of the Americas, New York, NY 10020

Natow, Annette B.
    The fat attack plan / Annette Natow, Jo-Ann Heslin.
        p.   cm.
    Includes bibliographical references.
    ISBN 0-671-68979-7: $18.95
    1. Reducing diets.   2. Low-fat diet.   I. Heslin, Jo-Ann.
II. Title.
RM222.2.N374   1990   89-49653
613.2'6–dc20   CIP

First Pocket Books hardcover printing April 1990

10   9   8   7   6   5   4   3   2   1

To our families, who support us through every project:
Harry, Allen, Irene, Sarah, Laura, Marty, George,
Emily, Steven, Joseph, Kristen, and Karen.

Acknowledgments

Our thanks to Dr. Irene Rosenberg for reviewing the material. Also to Dr. Martin Lefkowitz for his generosity in sharing resources. We also thank our clients and students, from whom we have learned so much. A special thanks to our agent, Nancy Trichter; Irwyn Applebaum; Claire Zion, our editor; and the production and publicity departments of Pocket Books.

"To eat out of proportion to one's need, either on the side of meagerness or superfluity, is culpable."

—MARY SWARTZ ROSE, PH.D.
Feeding the Family
The Macmillan Company, 1919

Contents

Introduction   1

1. *Fat Is a Killer*
   WHY WE MUST ATTACK FAT   5

2. *Let's Face Fats*
   THE SCIENCE OF FAT IN FOODS   13

3. *The Fat Attack Plan*
   AN OVERVIEW OF THE PROGRAM   22

4. *Eat Yourself Thin*
   AN OVERVIEW OF LOW-FAT FOODS   29

5. *Pectin Power*
   A NATURAL DIET AID   39

6. *Targeting Your Weight and Your Health Risks*
   WHERE TO START ON THE FAT ATTACK PLAN   44

7. *Super Start* FAT ATTACK PLAN PHASE ONE   55
   Super Start MENUS   75
   Super Start FOOD LISTS   135

8. *Getting Ahead* FAT ATTACK PLAN PHASE TWO   142
   Getting Ahead MENUS AND WORKSHEETS   161
   Getting Ahead FOOD LISTS   221

9. *In Control* FAT ATTACK PLAN PHASE THREE   234
   In Control MENUS AND WORKSHEETS   247
   In Control FOOD LISTS   293
   The Fat Attack Plan Fat Counter   300

10. *In Control at the Supermarket*
    HOW TO SHOP WHEN YOU'RE ATTACKING YOUR FAT   327

11. *In Control in Your Kitchen*
   TIPS FOR LOW-FAT COOKING   336

12. *In Control When You're Eating Out*
   SELECTING LOW-FAT RESTAURANT FOOD   341

13. *The Picture of Health*
   HOW DO YOU LOOK?   346

   Bibliography   351

Introduction

Not long ago, we conducted a lunchtime seminar at the headquarters of a major Fortune 500 company. It was the first in a series of talks we would be giving there, and the auditorium filled quickly. Testing the microphone and checking our watches, we were filled not only with typical pre-lecture excitement but also with a special enthusiasm because we were working with a large corporation that had made a commitment to good health for its employees.

But if anyone had asked us what we were going to talk about, we would have said we weren't quite sure yet. Naturally, not knowing what you're going to say can be a serious occupational hazard for public speakers. But this was exactly as we had planned it. The topic of our talk was "Why Do *You* Want to Diet?" and our idea was to let the audience get things started.

The first hand that went up belonged to an attractive young woman who said she'd had two babies in less than four years and was desperate to get back down to her wedding-day weight. She needed a diet that would take off her extra thirty pounds and keep it off, one that would be easy to incorporate into her busy schedule as a working mother.

Next we called on a man in his fifties who'd just learned that his cholesterol was too high. He wasn't really overweight, but his doctor had advised him to lose five or ten pounds and to change his eating habits to help bring his cholesterol down to a safer level.

Then a trim-looking woman in the back caught our attention. She didn't want to lose weight, she explained, but she'd been growing more concerned about cancer and other diseases, and she wondered if there was a diet that could really help prevent any of them.

We looked at each other and nodded. It was our turn to talk now, and we knew exactly what to say. "We're going to give all of you the same advice," we said. *"Attack your fat."*

Our seminar was off and running. Not surprisingly, the Fortune 500 group we were addressing provided a good random sampling of today's typical diet and health concerns. What *did* come as a surprise to a lot of people there, however, was that the answer to so many of these concerns was the same: **To lose weight, lower your cholesterol, and minimize many major health risks, all you have to do is reduce the fat in your diet.**

As Registered Dietitians who offer nutrition counseling to both individuals and professional groups, we find ourselves delivering this message more and more frequently. While many of the people we counsel are concerned with weight loss, a growing number are watching their cholesterol level or their blood pressure as well as their weight. Some, on the other hand, simply want a more healthful diet for themselves and their families. So this is what we tell our workshops and our college classes, our husbands, our children, our friends—and ourselves. It's what we say in textbooks, magazines, and private sessions: If you eat less fat you'll *be* less fat, and you'll be healthier, too.

Did you know that even though Americans are eating fewer calories now than in the past, average body weight has gone *up?* In 1960 the average man weighed 165; the average woman, 139. In 1980 he weighed 172 and she weighed 145! Yet on average, today's men take in only 90 percent of their recommended calories; today's women, only 82 percent.

Puzzling, isn't it. If Americans are eating "less," why are so many of them still fat? It's because of *what* they're eating, not how much. They're eating too much fat. Harvard Medical School researchers who analyzed the way overweight people eat found that the more fat these people ate, the more fat they had on their bodies—regardless of the total number of calories they took in.

But there's more going on here than just weight gain. Research is telling us that eating fat makes us fat. But it's also telling us that eating less fat will make us healthier. In fact, the Surgeon General's 1988 groundbreaking report on nutrition and health in America reaffirmed this advice by stating that "the primary priority for dietary change is the recommendation to reduce intake of total fats." When you put it all together, what does it mean—that *being* fat is unhealthy? Or that *eating* fat *makes* us unhealthy?

It's both. The overweight that a high-fat diet leads to can aggravate or worsen diabetes, coronary heart disease, osteoarthritis, and gout, and can cause significant increases in blood pressure and cholesterol and triglyceride levels. It can even shorten your life. The high-fat diet itself increases your risk for all these ills and, most sobering of all, for many kinds of cancer.

Nobody wants to be overweight. And thin or stout, everyone would like to live a healthier and longer life. They can. We now know that you *can* lose weight, keep it off, and ward off serious or even life-threatening diseases just by reducing the amount of fat you eat—by attacking your fat.

The Fat Attack Plan isn't just a weight-loss diet; it's a way of eating that you can start today—and continue every day for the rest of your life. On the Fat Attack Plan, you'll lose weight now *and* reduce your risk for life-threatening diseases by watching such factors as your blood pressure, weight, and cholesterol and triglyceride levels. And it will help you live longer to enjoy your good health.

On the Fat Attack Plan, you don't have to count calories. **All you have to do is learn to identify foods containing fat and eat less of them.** Sound too simple, a little too good to be true? Well, the beauty of the Fat Attack Plan *is* its simplicity. The only thing you watch is the amount of fat you eat; there's nothing else to count or control on this three-phase program.

The first phase achieves a quick weight loss with the help of a completely natural appetite suppressant and starts to bring down your total blood cholesterol and blood glucose (sugar) levels. In the second phase you continue to lose weight, while your blood glucose, cholesterol, and triglycerides go down. (Or, if you want to be healthier but have only a little weight to lose, you can start right off with phase two.)

In the third phase you establish a pattern for a lifetime of healthy eating, maintaining your weight loss and lowering your risk for serious illnesses.

We know for a fact that the Fat Attack Plan works. Hundreds of our clients have proved it by successfully losing weight, keeping it off, and lowering their health risks as they follow the meal plans and eating tips we've put together for them. They've learned to make low-fat choices at home, in the supermarket, and in restaurants. They're eating healthier and feeling better, and so are their families.

Now *you* can prove that our plan works, as well—simply by following the very same advice: Attack your fat!

1 *Fat Is a Killer*
WHY WE MUST ATTACK FAT

Why do *you* want to diet? Do you want to lose weight? Do you want to look better, and feel better, too? Get back into the clothes you were wearing a year ago?

Or do you think maybe you should just *change* your diet? Is it time to pay more attention to what you eat every day—and take a hard look at what it might be doing to you? Maybe your doctor has told you that your cholesterol level is too high or that your blood pressure has gone up in the last few years—and that losing some weight will help?

On the other hand, maybe you feel fine and look pretty good. You have a lot of energy and no real health problems. But don't you want to keep it that way? Don't you want to do everything you can to help prevent stroke and major diseases such as cancer, diabetes, and heart disease?

It doesn't matter what *your* reason is because they're all good reasons —and when you think about it, they all apply to every one of us anyway: We all want to look better, feel better, be healthier, and live longer.

The exciting news is that we all *can*—and the best part is that you can achieve weight loss and improved health *at the same time.* And you can do it easily and enjoyably.

If you want to lose weight, wouldn't you rather do it on a program that won't ever leave you feeling hungry? Of course you would. How about a program that's flexible and allows plenty of room for *your* food preferences? A program that will teach you good dietary habits in such an effective way that they'll soon become second nature? A program on which you *can't* cheat because *no* foods are forbidden?

Sounds pretty good, doesn't it? Well, there's more. On this program, you'll also end up with lower cholesterol, lower blood pressure, and a lowered risk for many major illnesses, too.

No matter what you weigh now, no matter what your health risks, no matter why *you* want to diet, the answer is the same. And it's a simple one: *Reduce the fat in your diet.*

By keeping just this one thing—fat—under control, you can lose weight *and* provide yourself with untold health benefits. That's what the Fat Attack Plan is all about, and that's why it works for everyone. Targeting the fat in your diet—and attacking it—is the most effective way to get the extra fat off your body. And it's also the surest way to prevent a number of serious, possibly life-threatening diseases.

Think about it. What do the following medical facts have in common?

- Although the number of deaths due to **coronary heart disease** has actually declined in America over the past decade, this preventable illness is still the number one killer in our country, responsible for 1.25 million heart attacks and half a million deaths each year.
- Nearly a million new cases of **cancer** are diagnosed here every year, and in 1987 alone 500,000 people died from cancer. Close to half of those people died from cancers that might have been prevented, yet cancer remains the number two cause of death in America.
- It is estimated that as many as 11 million Americans have **diabetes** today, half of them undiagnosed.
- **Stroke** victims in this country number half a million each year, and of them only 350,000 survive. Today 2 million Americans are living with stroke-related disabilities.
- **Obesity**, a critical risk factor for most life-threatening diseases, affects 34 million Americans between the ages of twenty and seventy-four.

What one factor is common to all these critical disorders, which shorten the lives of so many members of our health-conscious society? Lack of research dollars? Inadequate medical care? Pollution? It's something far more basic: It's *fat*. Cancer, heart disease, stroke, diabetes, and obesity are directly affected by what you eat, and by how much you weigh. Moreover, researchers are finding almost every day that many more disorders are affected by the amount of fat we eat. The common tie that binds together all these life-threatening diseases, and many chronic illnesses as well, is too much fat—in your food, and on your body.

The Official Word

Extensive research conducted over the past several years at university medical centers, government laboratories, independent institutions, and private facilities, both in this country and abroad, has documented over and over again that the amount and type of fat you eat, as well as being overweight, have a direct impact on your health. We now know that a high-fat diet can increase your risk for cancer, coronary heart disease, stroke, hypertension, diabetes, high cholesterol, gallstones, and arthritis, and that being overweight can make the situation even worse.

This is serious stuff—and, to many people, surprising and confusing as well. Can something they've been eating all their lives really be doing them such damage? Damage they might not yet even see any evidence of, except, perhaps, for a few extra pounds? But the message is supported by research findings, by the recommendations of many well-respected health organizations, and most recently by the Surgeon General. In the 1988 *Surgeon General's Report on Nutrition and Health,* then Surgeon General C. Everett Koop stated that "the primary priority for dietary change is the recommendation to reduce intake of total fats."

The sad reality is that too much fat can do more than just make you sick—it can actually kill you. "Overweight is risking fate," says obesity specialist Dr. George A. Bray, director of the Pennington Biomedical Research Center in Baton Rouge, Louisiana. Not only does excessively fatty food itself lead to coronary heart disease, certain forms of cancer, and possibly diabetes, but fat calories are now known to convert rapidly into body fat, adding another dimension not just to your figure but to your risk profile as well.

But the Surgeon General and organizations such as the American Heart Association, the American Diabetes Association, and the American Cancer Society aren't just dispensing advice; they're offering hope. *The good news is that by reducing our fat intake, we now can exercise a significant measure of control over the following "silent" killers:*

HEART DISEASE

The federal government makes periodic studies of the food consumption and general health of representative samplings of the U.S. population. Data from the last two of these HANES (Health and Nutrition Examination Survey) studies, as well as from several other studies, show a strong association between obesity and cardiovascular disease. And although the high-fat diet that leads to obesity is in itself a threat to cardiac health, too much body fat is indeed a problem as well. There is even evidence, according to Dr. Per Björntorp, a professor of medicine at the University of Göteborg in Sweden, that excess abdominal fat is more often related to heart disease than fat stored elsewhere, such as on the hips or thighs. The activity of the hormones that break down fatty tissue and deposit it into the bloodstream is greater in the midsection, Dr. Björntorp has found, making the fat stored in your abdomen potentially more dangerous to your cardiovascular health than fat found elsewhere on your body. Fat in the midsection also puts you at greater risk for diabetes.

Losing weight and following a low-fat eating plan can each diminish your risk for heart attack and stroke. First of all, achieving and maintaining normal weight will statistically lower your risk, and ridding your midsection of extra fat will further protect your heart and reduce your risk for diabetes. Together, losing weight *and* removing excess fat from your diet will lower your serum cholesterol level, one of the most significant ways to reduce your risk factor for heart disease.

HIGH SERUM CHOLESTEROL

Regardless of body weight, high levels of cholesterol in the blood pose a serious threat to cardiovascular health, increasing the possibility of heart attack and stroke. We also know that a diet high in fat—particularly saturated fat—is directly related to high cholesterol levels. It's not surprising, then, that overweight people are twice as likely to have high serum cholesterol levels, thus putting them at greater risk for heart disease.

Losing weight and following a low-fat eating plan will lower serum cholesterol levels. In its 1986 position statement, "Dietary Guidelines for Healthy American Adults," the American Heart Association, in response to the large and growing body of scientific evidence linking diet to heart disease, recommended that Americans cut their fat intake by one-third as a means of improving their cardiovascular health.

CANCER

The American Council of Science and Health reports that 20 to 25 percent of all Americans can expect to develop cancer at some point in their lives, and evidence now links both overweight *and* a high-fat diet—independent of each other—to increased prevalence of certain cancers. If you're an overweight man, you have a higher risk for death from cancer of the colon, rectum, or prostate. If you're an overweight woman, you have a higher risk for death from cancer of the breast, uterus, ovaries, gall bladder, or bile duct. And if you're a woman who's overweight *and* postmenopausal, your risk for breast cancer is even greater.

Eating too much fat, on the other hand, has been shown to independently increase the risk for breast, prostate, and colon cancer. In 1989, citing a study he had recently conducted in Italy, Dr. Paolo Taniolo of New York University's Medical Center reported that women who ate large amounts of fat had a risk for breast cancer that was three times greater than those who did not, and concluded that if you eat less fat you can reduce your risk for breast cancer.

Both a low-fat diet and weight loss may help prevent these three forms of cancer. The American Cancer Society's nutrition guidelines underscore this, with recommendations to "avoid obesity" and "cut down on total fat intake."

DIABETES

Diabetes is almost three times as likely in overweight people, and the risk for diabetes increases as body weight does. Moreover, the risk for heart disease is double in diabetic men and triple in diabetic women. We now know that obesity slightly alters body chemistry, reducing the body's ability to utilize insulin and thus promoting the development of diabetes. Some new evidence even suggests that a high-fat diet may clog the capillaries in the pancreas, where insulin is secreted, thus impairing the insulin production and activity necessary to maintain normal glucose (blood sugar) levels.

Maintaining normal body weight and cutting excess fat out of the diet can help prevent diabetes, or normalize it (by bringing blood sugar levels closer to normal). In fact, because blood sugar levels automatically drop when you eat less, it's possible for diabetics to see an improvement even before they've lost a noticeable amount of weight. The American, British, and Canadian diabetes associations all advise diabetics to "eat less fat" and maintain a normal body weight. And although it's true that persons with a family history of diabetes are more likely to develop it, their risk *can* be minimized by preventing or reversing overweight by means of a low-fat diet.

HYPERTENSION

Fifty-eight million Americans have high blood pressure, another disorder that the overweight are more likely to suffer: five times as likely if they're between the ages of twenty and forty-five, and twice as likely if they're between forty-five and seventy-five.

Exactly how weight gain causes high blood pressure is unknown, but we do know that **even modest weight loss causes a drop in blood pressure**. A low-fat diet will help achieve the weight loss so critical to hypertensives.

HIGH TRIGLYCERIDES

Triglycerides, like cholesterol, are all-important blood lipids (fats) that are measured to help determine risk for heart disease. Because of high-fat diets, overweight people are more likely to have hypertriglyceridemia—high levels of triglycerides in the blood—which, regardless of weight, may increase the risk for heart attack and stroke, particularly in postmenopausal women.

Weight loss and weight maintenance will often normalize high triglyceride levels, particularly by means of a low-fat diet, which will also lower other blood fats such as cholesterol.

ARTHRITIS

Osteoarthritis, a sometimes painful disease brought on by typical wear and tear on body joints, is known to be aggravated by overweight, which places additional burdens and strain on the entire body. **Losing weight can help ease the strain of arthritis.**

GALLSTONES

More than 15 percent of all Americans will develop gallstones at some point in their lifetime, and there is now clear evidence to show not only that eating a high-fat, high-cholesterol diet increases the likelihood of such stones, but also that overweight can be a contributing factor, independent of diet. Data collected from the Framingham Study, a long-term population study of diet and health risks in one Massachusetts city, show a connection between gallstones and both obesity and high-fat diets. Although we've learned that women are twice as likely to suffer from gallstones as men are, the heavier a person gets the more likely he or she is to develop gallstones, regardless of sex.

A low-fat diet, which automatically means reduced intake of cholesterol as well as weight loss, will help decrease the risk for developing gallstones.

GOUT

People who weigh too much or eat too much fat are more prone to gout, the deposit of uric acid crystals in the small joints of the body. These crystals are more likely to form when uric acid levels in the blood are high, a condition aggravated by a high-fat diet, which slows the normal elimination of uric acid from the body. Gout can be painful, disfiguring, and disabling.

A low-fat diet aids in the elimination of uric acid and promotes the weight loss essential to reducing the risk for and incidence of gout.

RESPIRATORY PROBLEMS

Overweight places an extra burden on every body system. But as a person becomes heavier and fat accumulates around the chest area, lung and diaphragm movement is impaired, and breathing often becomes more difficult. This not only puts a strain on the heart, but also aggravates or worsens respiratory problems such as influenza, pneumonia, and obstructive lung disease—illnesses that can ultimately lead to death. **Weight loss can alleviate breathing difficulties.**

DIGESTIVE PROBLEMS

Have you ever eaten a meal that was delicious but seemingly indigestible? It probably had too much fat in it. Fat takes longer to leave your stomach than protein and carbohydrates do, so a high-fat meal can leave you with an uncomfortable, bloated feeling and an upset stomach. And when food moves more slowly through your digestive tract, the bacteria there have more opportunity to ferment it, thus causing extra gas as well.

Overweight people often feel these problems more acutely than those who maintain normal weight. Extra fat around the abdomen can put pressure on the stomach, forcing its contents back up into the esophagus and causing heartburn and discomfort.

Low-fat foods are easier on the stomach, and will promote the weight loss that contributes to better digestion.

Obesity, Life-span, and the Fat Attack Plan

We've seen now what a great number of serious, sometimes life-threatening illnesses are influenced by overweight and by the rich, fatty foods that lead to overweight. **At all ages, people who are fatter are more likely to die, because obesity shortens your life-span.** Fat *is* a killer. But you can turn the whole situation around simply by eating less fat.

Naturally, a lot of the people who come to us for advice are primarily interested in losing weight. But as we counsel these people through the phases of their weight loss, they learn that by losing weight *and* eating less fat they're really getting a package deal: They end up looking better, and they end up a lot healthier, too. With the help of the Fat Attack Plan, they actually give themselves a good chance of escaping the life-threatening medical problems that everyone would like to avoid.

If that's what you'd like to do, too, you've come to the right place.

Whether you're interested in losing weight, lowering your health risks, discovering a better way of eating, or all three, you can—simply by following the Fat Attack Plan.

Remember, the *only* thing you have to do is learn to recognize the fat in your diet—and attack it! And that's exactly what the Fat Attack Plan will teach you to do, because it's a *learning* plan. As you read from chapter to chapter, and as your own fat attack progresses from phase to phase, you'll learn all about fat and how to attack it by adopting a healthy new way of eating. By the time you've reached your target weight you'll have all the tools you need for a lifetime of good low-fat eating—and good health, too.

In chapter 2 you'll learn just what fat is, why it makes you fat, and how to find it in the foods you eat. Then, in chapter 3, which presents the three different phases of the Fat Attack Plan, you'll get a complete overview of the program and what each different phase can do.

Chapter 4 will teach you about all the low-fat foods that will help you attack your fat: the delicious, healthy fruits, vegetables, grains, legumes, and low-fat dairy and protein foods that you'll be basing your new eating plan on—the foods that will help you "eat yourself thin." Best of all, we're going to make it even easier for you to lose weight and reduce your health risks. How? With the help of a completely natural diet aid that's truly good for you. You'll learn all about this "hunger chaser" in chapter 5.

Once you have the basics, where do you begin? Well, to help you determine which phase of the Fat Attack Plan you should start with, chapter 6 offers a Health Risks Quiz and several methods of determining the correct, healthy weight for you. Once you know what your risks are —if any—and how much you should weigh, you'll be able to pinpoint right away just where to begin your own personal fat attack.

Sound good? Then to keep first things first, let's take a look at fat itself. If you're going to attack it, you have to understand what it is and know where to find it. Good luck! You're on your way to good looks—and good health!

2 *Let's Face Fats*
THE SCIENCE OF FAT IN FOODS

One of the most challenging aspects of our role as nutrition counselors is keeping abreast of current scientific information about diet, nutrition, and health, and then carefully translating it into safe and workable advice for our clients. While some of the studies we read about confirm established fact, others yield fresh nuances that prompt researchers to look in new directions. This endless "search and discovery" is part of what makes the scientific process so fascinating.

But it's also what makes translating this data correctly one of the most critical things we do. We all know how easy it is to be confused or even misled by what we read or hear, particularly when a new research finding is announced in the media. That's why guarding against misinterpretation of new information and presenting established information clearly are so important to us. Teaching our clients well is the best way we know to help them help themselves.

While this is always our aim, it seems even more important when we are helping people establish and maintain low-fat eating habits because this kind of advice isn't temporary. We're teaching a whole new way of healthy eating and living. During the past five years alone, we've seen such a dramatic increase in the amount of scientific evidence that isolates reducing fat intake as the best means of promoting better health, there's no longer any question that this is the way to go.

That's why we created the Fat Attack Plan and designed it in such a way that it teaches you as you go along. When you follow the preplanned "Super Start" and "Getting Ahead" menus you'll automatically be eating less fat (but you'll always get more than enough to meet your body's needs). You'll also be learning how to make sensible fat choices. By the time you're in the third phase, "In Control," you'll be making all these choices on your own. The *only* thing you'll ever have to watch by the time you're "In Control" is the total amount of fat in the food you eat: forty-five grams a day if you're a woman, sixty grams a day if you're a man.

In addition to knowing which foods contain fat, and how much, we think it's also useful to know a little about fat itself. While you certainly don't have to become an expert in the chemistry of fat in order to be slim and healthy, knowing the basics about this dietary element and its effect on the human body will help you understand why the Fat Attack Plan works as well as it does.

What Should You Know About Fat?

You're probably already familiar with the three types of dietary fat: saturated, polyunsaturated, and monounsaturated. You see these names on margarine packages and salad oil labels, hear them mentioned in advertisements, and read about them in newspaper and magazine articles all the time. But how are they different from one another? And is any one of them better or worse for you than the others?

Let's start with some basics. Chemically, all fats are combinations of fatty acids (carbon atoms holding hydrogen atoms) and glycerol (an alcohol). The terms *saturated, polyunsaturated,* and *monounsaturated* refer to the chemical structure of the fatty acids. In a saturated fatty acid, all the carbon atoms are holding as many hydrogen atoms as they can. In a monounsaturated fatty acid, two carbon atoms are each missing one hydrogen atom. In a polyunsaturated fatty acid, four or more carbon atoms are missing hydrogen atoms.

But it's important to understand that no dietary fats—fat foods—are made exclusively of one kind of fatty acid; in fact, they're all mixtures of all three. For example, olive oil is called a monounsaturated fat, but that's only because it's *primarily* monounsaturated. It also contains small amounts of polyunsaturated and saturated fatty acids. Safflower oil, on the other hand, is called a polyunsaturated fat because it contains more "polys" than other kinds of fatty acids.

SATURATED FATS

Saturated fats are the kind that stay solid at room temperature. A good example of saturated fat is the fat around a chop or steak. Even if you left the meat on the kitchen counter for several hours, the fat would still be solid.

Saturated fats are generally found in animal products, such as meat, milk, cheese, and butter. But some vegetable products—notably the "tropical" oils (coconut, palm, and palm kernel) and cocoa butter—are highly saturated as well. (Vegetable products can even be made more saturated, and thus firmer, through a process called hydrogenation. This is how corn oil is turned into margarine.)

Studies have shown that most saturated fats raise levels of both HDL (high-density lipoprotein, or "good") cholesterol, and LDL (low-density lipoprotein, or "bad") cholesterol in the blood. This is why we've been urged to curtail our intake of saturated fats.

But a study completed recently at the Southwestern Medical School of the University of Texas has shown that not all saturated fats raise cholesterol after all. Beef, for example, contains not only polyunsaturated and monounsaturated fats as well as the saturated fat for which it is known, but also several *different* saturated fats, among them palmitic fatty acid (which raises cholesterol) and stearic fatty acid (which lowers it).

Current recommendations suggest that saturated fats make up no more than one-third of your total fat intake each day. But as a practical matter, of course, where saturated fat is concerned it would be impossible to choose only foods with those saturated fatty acids that lower cholesterol. As more research is done, the findings sometimes seem to get more confusing. It's much simpler and just as effective to limit your intake of fats in general, since all fat foods are combinations of fatty acids anyway.

POLYUNSATURATED FATS

Polyunsaturated fats are liquid at room temperature and remain liquid even when cold. If, for example, you put a bottle of safflower oil in the refrigerator and left it there all day, it would still remain liquid.

Polyunsaturated fats are the main fatty acid found in vegetable oils, such as corn, cottonseed, sunflower, safflower, and soybean oils. While "polys" are known to reduce the "bad" LDLs, they also reduce the "good" HDLs. Some new research also indicates that there may be other harmful effects associated with them, such as increased risk for cancer, gallstone formation, and suppression of immune function.

Fish contains a unique kind of polyunsaturated fat, known as EPA (eicosapentanoic acid) or DHA (docosahexanoic) acid. Often popularly referred to as "Omega-3" fatty acids (so named because of their chemical structure), these fats are found in larger amounts in fatty cold-water fish (such as salmon, mackerel, bluefish, herring, squid, rainbow trout, and whitefish) than in lean fish (like cod and halibut).

Omega-3s are currently under careful study, for they may benefit rheumatoid arthritis, immune function, high blood pressure, psoriasis, and migraine headaches. They seem to reduce the risk for the abnormal clotting that may lead to heart attacks and strokes, and they do lower triglyceride levels in the blood. Yet many experts feel that more research is needed before a recommendation can be made about the specific value of fish oil in the human diet. Nevertheless, while the current recommendation for consumption of all polyunsaturated fats in general is that they be limited to less than one-third of our total fat intake, it's a good practice to make foods rich in Omega-3s part of this total.

MONOUNSATURATED FATS

"Monos" are liquid at room temperature, but may become solid when cold. Olive oil is perhaps the best example of a monounsaturated fat; kept in the cupboard it remains clear and liquid, but stored in the refrigerator it may become cloudy and begin to solidify.

Olives and olive oil, canola (rapeseed) oil, peanuts and peanut oil, walnuts and walnut oil, sesame seeds, sesame oil, and tahini (sesame paste), as well as chicken fat and solid vegetable shortening all contain large amounts of monounsaturated fats.

Research has shown that when "monos" are substituted for the saturated fats in our diet, blood cholesterol may be lowered. The special value of these fats, moreover, is that they seem to selectively lower only the harmful form of cholesterol (LDL) but not the beneficial form (HDL). This is why current recommendations suggest that *more than one-third of your daily fat intake come from monounsaturated fats.*

What Kind of Fat Should You Eat?

The current recommendation for daily fat intake is:

- more than one-third monounsaturated
- less than one-third saturated
- less than one-third polyunsaturated

While it is important to change the kinds of fat you eat, it's not an easy job to choose foods that supply the recommended levels of saturated, polyunsaturated, and monounsaturated fats. As a general rule it makes sense to substitute vegetable oils (like corn or olive oil) for animal and dairy fats (like butter) and to eat fish and chicken instead of red meat whenever you can. Try, too, to avoid lard, tropical oils, and cocoa butter (which is found in chocolate).

But you don't need to worry about this too much now. The food choices in the Fat Attack Plan emphasize these sensible alternatives, and following the program will help you learn to make good fat choices. And, you can also get an idea of the fat components of some familiar foods by looking at the following list. Just remember: Don't lose sight of the bigger picture in an attempt to substitute one fat for another. It's much simpler just to remember to eat *less* fat; specific fat reduction will then take care of itself. You'll lose weight and be even healthier for reducing your overall fat intake.

WHAT'S THE DIFFERENCE
BETWEEN FAT AND CHOLESTEROL?

In the wake of all the discussion about fat and cholesterol these days, it might seem easy to confuse the two, particularly since some foods contain both. But fat and cholesterol aren't the same at all.

Fat, like protein and carbohydrates, provides calories—fuel for your body to run on. Cholesterol, on the other hand, is a fatlike substance that's found in foods of animal origin only, foods such as meat, poultry, fish, and dairy products. It's possible to have a food that's high in fat but low in cholesterol, like the new butter-margarine blends. It's also possible to have a food that's low in fat but high in cholesterol, like an egg.

Cholesterol is not an essential nutrient that must be obtained from food. But it is an important part of our cell membranes, and it's naturally present in all our cells already because the human body actually makes all the cholesterol it needs.

Cholesterol (whether it comes from food you eat or is manufactured by your body) travels through your body in your bloodstream; thus, the term "blood cholesterol" (or "serum cholesterol") is used to describe the level of cholesterol in your blood. But because of its waxy nature, cholesterol can't dissolve in blood, which is mostly water. Instead, it's transported by special "lipoprotein carriers," little packages of fat wrapped in water-soluble protein.

Although there are several different kinds of carriers, the ones you're most likely to hear about are "LDLs" (low-density lipoproteins) and "HDLs" (high-density lipoproteins). LDLs are often called "bad cholesterol" because the cholesterol in LDLs can end up on your artery walls. HDLs, on the other hand, are sometimes referred to as "good cholesterol" because they carry cholesterol back to the liver, where it is broken down and removed from the body.

Why Is Fat So Fattening?

We've already learned how serious the health consequences of a high-fat diet can be; that, in fact, excess fat in your diet and on your body can actually kill you. Now let's take a look at why the extra fat in your diet shows up so quickly on your body.

For years we've heard that people get fat simply because they eat more food than they need. Take in too many calories every day and you'll put on a few pounds in no time. Well, that's true—sort of. But we now know that it depends on the *kinds* of calories you eat, because strange as it

FAT DISTRIBUTION IN COMMON FOODS

Food	Polyunsaturated	Saturated	Monounsaturated
Cheddar cheese	3.0%	59.0%	38.0%
Creamed cottage cheese	—	50.0%	50.0%
Whole egg, large	8.0%	35.5%	56.5%
Butter	2.5%	57.5%	40.0%
Corn oil	51.0%	12.0%	37.0%
Margarine, stick	10.0%	27.5%	62.5%
Lean fish	19.0%	16.0%	65.0%
Lamb, leg, untrimmed	5.5%	63.5%	31.0%
Pork loin, untrimmed	9.0%	36.0%	55.0%
Sirloin, untrimmed	3.0%	46.0%	51.0%
Veal, chuck, untrimmed	—	45.0%	55.0%
Ice cream	—	56.0%	44.0%
Peanuts	18.0%	14.0%	68.0%
Chicken, with skin	19.0%	40.0%	41.0%

may sound at first, all calories are not created equal. Where gaining and losing weight are concerned, a calorie from a stalk of broccoli just isn't the same as a calorie from a pat of butter.

Why? First and most important, the fat in foods is very similar in chemical composition to the fat on our bodies. It doesn't take much effort at all for our bodies to turn dietary fat right into body fat and store it away for future energy use, since turning food fat into body fat uses up only 3 percent of all the calories in the fat. Carbohydrate (sugar and starch) and protein calories, on the other hand, which are usually burned immediately for energy, are harder to convert; in fact, at least 23 percent of the carbohydrate calories you eat are burned up in the conversion process!

Second, fat foods are frighteningly high in calories. Weight for weight, fat has more than twice as many calories (nine per gram) as protein or carbohydrates (which each have four per gram). So even a little bit of butter on your bagel is going to raise the calorie count quite a bit—and with the kind of calories that can quickly end up in the wrong place. And, interestingly, high-fat diets *seem* to make you eat more: Although researchers aren't sure why it happens, their repeated observations have shown that people on high-fat diets simply eat more food.

Given these facts it's not hard to understand why people who eat more fat *are* more fat, and why the Fat Attack Plan will help you lose weight readily, keep it off, and become healthier at the same time.

Do we need any fat at all? Yes. Our bodies need some fat called essential fatty acids to function normally. Fat is also needed to transport vitamins and to provide some padding for our internal organs. And we know that fats make food taste good. It's not that you should never eat another slice of cheese—on the Fat Attack Plan you'll learn to make fat food choices every day—it's just that the amount of fat Americans eat on average (as much as 40 percent of their daily calories are from fat) is far more than they need.

Rating Your Fat Intake

This is a good time to see how much fat there is in your own diet by taking the following quiz.

1. I use butter or margarine at most meals.   Yes   No
2. I lighten my coffee or tea with cream, half-and-half (light cream), or non-dairy creamers.   Yes   No
3. I eat cheese four or more times a week.   Yes   No
4. I use regular sour cream or cream cheese four or more times a week.   Yes   No
5. I drink whole milk.   Yes   No
6. I eat meat, fish, or poultry every day.   Yes   No
7. Most days I eat bacon, sausage, or luncheon meat.   Yes   No
8. I eat fried or breaded food three or more times a week.   Yes   No
9. I usually eat foods with sauce or gravy.   Yes   No
10. I usually eat salads with regular dressing or mayonnaise.   Yes   No
11. I rarely eat fresh fruits and vegetables.   Yes   No
12. I eat in a fast-food restaurant every week.   Yes   No
13. I eat ice cream, pie, or cake for dessert three or more times a week.   Yes   No
14. I snack on chocolate, chips, or nuts.

Every "yes" says "too much fat," and increases your chance of being too fat—*and* your risk for heart disease, cancer, and other serious health problems. But don't be discouraged. As you progress through the Fat Attack Plan, come back every so often and take the quiz again. Your goal, of course, is to reduce your "Yes" answers to as few as possible—

ultimately to no more than one at most. And while this may seem like a tough goal now, you'll probably be surprised at how quickly "Yes" turns to "No" once you're on the Fat Attack Plan.

It's Everywhere

Just as most people are surprised to learn how many health problems are caused by an excess of fat in their diet, they're also surprised to learn that fat lurks in so many of the foods they've been eating for years—foods like the ones on the quiz you just took. For while some fats are visible (obvious things like butter and margarine or the fat on a piece of bacon), fat is also present even if you can't see it. Nuts, seeds, cheese, milk, pastries, muffins, and salad dressings all contain fat. Even breads, cereals, vegetables, and some fruits contain traces of fat. Let's take a closer look at all these foods to see where the fat is.

FATS AND OILS

It's likely that about one-third of your daily fat intake comes from pure fats and oils: vegetable shortening, butter or margarine, and olive or other vegetable oils. These fats are easy to identify in your diet—which also makes them easy to remove.

MEATS, FISH, POULTRY

Most of us get more than one-fourth of our fat each day from meat, fish, and poultry. It's easy to see and cut off some of the fat from steaks, chops, and even poultry and some fish. (Bacon has so much visible fat that we can hardly call it meat.)

But all of these protein foods also have "invisible" fat found in pockets throughout the flesh—fat which can't be trimmed away because it's part of the structure of the flesh itself. The amount of fat in this group of foods varies dramatically: Beef and pork hot dogs, luncheon meats, sausages, prime ribs, mackerel, salmon, and duck have much more fat than other choices such as flank steak, sirloin tip, cod, halibut, skinless turkey or chicken breast, and chicken or turkey franks.

DAIRY FOODS

While many calcium-rich dairy foods—like milk, yogurt, ice cream, and cheese—now come in "regular," "reduced-fat," and even "nonfat" varieties, if you choose the regular variety you could easily end up getting as much as one-fifth of your daily fat from them. Regular sour cream and cream cheese are extremely high in fat, as are cream, "gourmet" ice cream, and most hard cheeses, like cheddar (which you really should consider a fat food, not a protein). You can easily reduce some of the fat in these foods by choosing the low-fat or, if available, the nonfat versions.

HIDDEN FATS

Then there are those foods we've learned about that contain a lot of fat or oil, like mayonnaise or potato chips. But if you dig a little deeper into the typical American diet you'll see that there's fat—often a lot—in many other things: cookies, doughnuts and pastries, granola, non-dairy creamers, breaded and fried foods, sauces and gravies, soups and stews, salad dressings, nuts, candy bars, and even avocados and olives. Eating anything prepared with added or hidden fats (which are frequently found in prepackaged foods) is going to boost your daily fat intake considerably.

Attack Your Fat

The solution, of course, is to make sensible food choices—cutting the excess fat out of your diet while enjoying healthy, satisfying meals and snacks. That's exactly what so many of our clients have done by following the Fat Attack Plan, and you can do the same: lose weight, reduce your risk for serious illness, and get started on a program of good eating for a lifetime of good health. Ready? **Attack your fat!**

3 *The Fat Attack Plan*
AN OVERVIEW OF THE PROGRAM

Researchers have uncovered a lot of the secrets of nutrition science in the past several years. They've helped make our job easier in some ways and more challenging in others. But one thing that's never been a secret is the fact that all dieters want a delicious, easy-to-follow plan that will help them lose weight quickly without going hungry. They admit that their diet should be a nutritious one, but most of all they just never want to see those extra pounds again. They simply want to be thinner—although they never complain when they also end up healthier.

It's our job to help them be both. Many of our clients come to us with other special health concerns that can be helped—or hindered—by what they eat. So even before we had the answers we now have to questions like "What makes us fat?" and "What foods are healthiest?" we were working hard to create balanced, appetizing meals for people who needed to lose weight as well as for people who didn't.

So we've always had more than weight loss in mind. But as time went on and research continued to provide us with additional data, we found ourselves offering more and more of our clients the same advice, regardless of why they had come to us. We'd tell them to reduce the fat in their diet.

That's why we created the Fat Attack Plan, because it's the one answer to a lot of very important questions, like "What's the best way to lose weight and keep it off?" and "How can I stay healthy and live longer?"

A Way of Eating, Not a Diet

Most people think of a diet as something they follow to lose weight. But the Fat Attack Plan is more than that kind of diet. Yes, you'll lose weight if that's your goal; but far more important, you'll learn a whole new way of healthy, low-fat eating. The Fat Attack Plan will help you lose weight now, reduce your risk for major illnesses, and increase your chance of living a longer, healthier life.

We know fat has to go. Too much of it not only ruins our appearance, but it raises our cholesterol and can also make us very, very sick. Bluntly stated, fat is a direct route to many of the life-threatening diseases that we don't even want to think about, much less get.

So we attacked it. Armed with all the new findings about fat, and relying on our combined three decades of training and experience, we designed a delicious, healthy three-phase plan that contains enough—but not too much—fat. It's a plan that will teach you how to keep your intake of fat at a safe level. **On the Fat Attack Plan, the only thing you have to do is learn to identify foods that contain fat and eat less of them. There are no other limits.** You'll simply learn to spot the fat in all the foods you're familiar with, and you'll be able to eat all those foods, in appropriate amounts.

We'll help you make some of your food choices at first, if that's what you want. Or you can design many of your meals yourself. In a short time you'll be doing it *all* on your own: making sensible fat choices from foods you like and enjoying many other delicious low-fat foods as well. We'll show you how.

A Three-Phase Plan

No matter what you want to achieve—a svelte new shape or a cholesterol cure, a thirty-five-pound makeover or just ten pounds off in time for your class reunion—you can tailor your "Fat Attack" to your own needs. If you want to lose weight, you will—with the help of a completely natural diet aid we call a "hunger chaser" because it will "chase your hunger" away. And if you need to lower your cholesterol or your other risk factors for serious diseases, you can do that, too. When we created the Fat Attack Plan we did it with a lot of different people in mind.

That's why it's presented in three different phases: "Super Start," "Getting Ahead," and "In Control." In "Super Start," weight loss is the target. "Getting Ahead" lowers your cholesterol and brings your weight down, too. When you're "In Control," you'll be maintaining your weight, your lowered cholesterol, and your overall good health.

Targeting Your Weight Goals and Health Risks

We all want to be healthier. Some of us want to be healthier *and* thinner. But how do you know which phase of the Fat Attack Plan to start with? That all depends on what your weight goals and health needs are.

The first thing you'll do is determine what weight is best for your specific body size and type with the help of the weight tables in chapter 6. Next you'll take a quick quiz to determine your health risks, if any.

You'll review your family history for illnesses, such as cancer, diabetes, and heart disease, then answer some questions about your own health, taking a look at your weight, blood pressure, and cholesterol and triglyceride levels. Then you'll learn a little about what your answers mean.

Once you've targeted your weight and health risks, you'll know where to start. If you need to lose twelve to twenty-five pounds and want to reduce your health risks, you'll begin with "Super Start" and then move into "Getting Ahead." If you need to lose only five to fourteen pounds and want to reduce your health risks, you can jump right into "Getting Ahead." If you have more than twenty-five pounds to lose and need to reduce your health risks, you'll do it by alternating "Super Start" and "Getting Ahead" until you've reached your goal.

If you have no weight to lose, or if you've reached your weight-loss goal, you'll follow "In Control" for a sound program of delicious low-fat eating and a longer, healthier life.

Even without consulting the weight tables or reviewing your "vital numbers," you may already have an idea of where you should begin your Fat Attack. Let's take a closer look at each of the three phases to see what they have to offer you and how they work.

"Super Start"

If you begin your Fat Attack with Super Start, you'll be surprised at how much better you'll feel almost immediately, and you'll see rapid, substantial weight loss. This is the phase to get you going if you want to lose twelve to fifteen pounds now, or a total of twenty-five pounds or more by the time you're "In Control." Super Start features preplanned menus that you can follow "as is," or you can repeat the same menus over and over if that's what appeals to you. It doesn't matter, because all the breakfasts are nutritionally equivalent, as are all the lunches and all the dinners.

You'll eat less fat in Super Start than in any of the other Fat Attack phases, but that's what will help you achieve such quick, noticeable results. What *will* you eat? Lots of nutritious, low-fat foods, such as lean meat, poultry and fish, cereals, breads and grains, vegetables, fruits, salads, and low-fat dairy products.

You'll get lots of snacks, too—even wine, if that's what you choose. There are recipes for delicious low-fat meals, and you'll learn a host of new cooking ideas for preparing your food without added fat.

You'll start learning about low-fat food choices. That's one of the great things about the Fat Attack Plan—you learn as you go, and by the time you're In Control you'll be an expert on low-fat eating. You'll also learn that even if you can't make ideal choices *all* the time, your weight loss won't go down the drain as long as you're making them most of the time.

YOUR NATURAL "HUNGER CHASER"

Although some people tell us there's almost too much food on Super Start, most of our clients are thrilled to find out that they can help themselves along with a completely natural diet aid: powdered pectin. This is a fiber made from apples and grapefruit, and when it's added to food it makes you feel full longer. That's why we call it a "hunger chaser." On Super Start, you can add powdered pectin to your food at lunch and at dinner (we'll show you exactly what to do in chapter 7). You'll never taste the difference, but your stomach won't empty as fast, and you'll feel satisfied longer.

"Getting Ahead"

If losing five to fourteen pounds and lowering your health risks are what you're after, Getting Ahead is the place for *you* to start. This Fat Attack phase targets lowering your cholesterol, triglycerides, blood sugar, and weight.

Like Super Start, Getting Ahead offers twenty-eight days of low-fat, fiber-rich cereals, vegetables, fruits, salads, grains, and breads, as well as lean meat, fish and poultry, and low-fat dairy foods. But you'll also be choosing fifteen grams of fat yourself from a long list of fat choices and adding them to your meal plans each day. This will help you learn more about making sensible fat choices and how to track the fat in your diet.

The first fourteen days of Getting Ahead offer preplanned menus; but foods are interchangeable, so you can stick with your favorites if you want to. In addition to your fat choices, you'll be able to choose from Main Dishes and Side Dishes at dinner. Then, on the fifteenth day, you'll begin to make all your food choices yourself, with the help of a simple outline of the Getting Ahead eating plan.

"In Control"

When you're "In Control," you're just that: in control of all your food choices. This third phase of the Fat Attack Plan is a flexible, lifelong plan for healthy eating that will maintain your weight, keep your cholesterol and other health risks down, and make you feel terrific! The only thing you'll have to do is watch the amount of fat you eat: no more than forty-five grams a day if you're a woman, or sixty grams a day if you're a man —the right amount for good health.

If you start out with Super Start or Getting Ahead, by the time you're In Control tracking your fat will be second nature. Even if you have no weight to lose and start out "In Control," you'll get the hang of it in no time. Tracking fat is a lot easier than counting calories—there's less to count, and many foods are fat free. Our "Fat Counter," which tells you just how much fat there is in hundreds of the foods we all like to eat, makes it even easier.

You'll build your daily menus on a basic eating plan that outlines the recommended number of servings of all the good foods that contribute to a balanced diet: fruits; vegetables; breads, cereals, and grains; low-fat dairy foods; and lean meats, poultry, and fish. While some of your daily fat intake will come from these foods, most of them are fat free, so you'll find there's plenty of room to personalize your diet with the fat choices you do make. We'll even give you sample menus for both men and women, including suggestions for fast-food meals, social occasions, and enjoying the special foods you love—all while you're "In Control."

And to help make your new eating plan even easier for you and your family to follow, we'll take a trip to the supermarket together for a lesson in label reading and smart, low-fat shopping. Then we'll show you how to keep things "In Control" in your kitchen and give you some solid advice on healthy, enjoyable restaurant eating.

THE "FAT ATTACK TARGET"

The "Fat Attack Target" is a great reference tool for keeping "In Control." On the target, which you can take a peek at on page 241, we've organized several basic fat foods in such a way that you can tell at a glance which you should eat less of because they're high in fat, and which you can eat more of because they're lower in fat. The "Fat Attack Target" also shows you which foods you don't even have to worry about because they're so low in fat that they're "free." Our clients find this handy visual aid helpful, and we think you will, too: You can make a copy to carry with you, or even stick it on your refrigerator with a magnet.

Doing Our Homework

The Fat Attack Plan is based on a research program we conducted during a sabbatical from Adelphi University in New York. The goal of our program was to help a group of overweight adults lose weight and reduce severe risk for heart disease and diabetes. Every one of our subjects had tried to do these things before, but they had been unsuccessful; in fact, many of them entered our study because the only other alternative was to take medication for their conditions.

In this research group, every one of our subjects lost weight on the low-fat eating plan we designed for them, and most of them substantially reduced their risk for heart disease and diabetes as well. They also lowered their cholesterol, their blood glucose, and their triglycerides. To our delight, research conducted in many other settings throughout the United States has validated our findings. By reinforcing and adding to our nutrition knowledge, this research has helped us develop the Fat Attack Plan.

Sometimes research tells us exactly what we think it will; other times we get surprises. One interesting and important finding that came out of our study was that several well-educated people who considered themselves knowledgeable about nutrition weren't able to translate their knowledge into practice. What we discovered was that although they wanted to know about eating right, much of their knowledge was incomplete and simply reflected popular, oftentimes half-true messages delivered by the media.

When asked how they could eat less fat, for example, many in this group suggested switching from butter to margarine, not realizing that, weight for weight, butter and margarine have the same amount of fat. Most likely they assumed that margarine has less fat than butter because of the way it's promoted: as being better for you than butter because it contains no cholesterol. Yet when they learned how to reduce their total fat intake by following the principles on the Fat Attack Plan, they lost weight and saw dramatic reductions in their health risks.

Something else a lot of people don't realize is that some weight-loss diets really aren't as healthy as they might seem to be at first. High-protein diets are a good example. Most of the foods we consider high in protein—such as meat, cheese, and milk—are also naturally high in fat, so eating a lot of these means you're taking in a lot of fat. Processing protein is also very hard work for your body, and getting rid of the waste products from protein can put a lot of stress on your kidneys. The far better course is a low-fat diet with the right amount of protein and lots of high-fiber, high-carbohydrate foods, such as vegetables, fruits, breads, cereals, and grains.

You'll learn all about these nutritious foods in chapter 4, where we'll teach you many of the same principles of low-fat living that we teach our clients and our classes. And of course, you'll continue to learn as you progress through your Fat Attack Plan. You'll probably even "un-learn" some incorrect things as well.

Untangling complex scientific information about anything is a job best left to the experts. But we all have to eat, and most people have a real interest in food. What happens, unfortunately, is that information about nutrition is often presented by people who haven't been trained in the science of nutrition. But our training—coupled with our "continuing education" and years of experience as translators of complicated information about foods and nutrition—is what enables us to teach, one of the most important things we do.

It's also what enabled us to create the Fat Attack Plan, present it to so many people, and help them make it work. We took all the facts and findings about fat and the body's use of it, and turned them into practical choices for weight loss and improved health. Now those same practical choices will help *you* lose weight, lower your health risks, and live longer. We did the homework, but you get the A!

STARTING YOUR FAT ATTACK

1. **Target your weight**: Determine what weight is best for your specific body size and type with the help of the weight tables on pages 48–49 in chapter 6.

2. **Target your health risks**: Take the quiz that starts on page 49 in chapter 6 to determine your health risks, if any.

3. **Determine where to start**: With the help of the information on pages 53–54 in chapter 6, pinpoint whether you should start your Fat Attack with Super Start, Getting Ahead, or In Control.

4 *Eat Yourself Thin*
AN OVERVIEW OF LOW-FAT FOODS

One of the very best things about the Fat Attack Plan—one of the most important things to learn—is that there are *no* forbidden foods. Not even fat foods! Our clients sometimes can't believe it when we tell them that once they're "In Control" they really can have some sour cream on their baked potato, or a hot fudge sundae once in a while if they're dying for one. Even the "Getting Ahead" phase, on which you'll lose weight and lower your cholesterol, includes a daily allowance of fifteen grams of fat that you get to choose.

It's all a matter of moderation, of course, and balance. The federal government's 1976–80 Health and Nutrition Examination Survey revealed that most American men were eating upwards of ninety-eight grams of fat a day, and women, about sixty. Unquestionably, there was far too much fat in those diets, and recent samplings show that things haven't changed. But when you're following a balanced eating plan like the Fat Attack Plan, one that's made up mostly of nutritious low-fat foods, there's room for some added fat.

You've already learned quite a bit about fat foods, and you'll learn a lot more as you move through the Fat Attack Plan—how to choose them sensibly and how to track the amount of fat they contain. But what about all the foods you *don't* have to track? The ones you get to enjoy without a second thought?

There's a whole world of "free foods" out there: breads, cereals, pastas, grains, fruits, vegetables, and beans. These high-carbohydrate foods contain very little or no fat at all, so there's nothing to track—and nothing to worry about—when you eat them. And eat them you will! You'll find an abundance of all these fat-free beauties in Super Start and Getting Ahead, and they'll play a central role in your balanced, nutritious In Control Menu Planner. These are the foods you need as your allies in order to attack your fat successfully, so we'll fully review them in this chapter. They're the foods that will help you "eat yourself thin."

The Fat Attack Plan—like any good eating plan, whether it's for losing or maintaining weight—contains a variety of foods from several different food groups. All three phases of the Fat Attack Plan are based on the low-fat, high-carbohydrate foods that provide top nourishment by fulfilling all your body's requirements for protein, fiber, vitamins, and minerals. They'll make you feel energetic, help you lose weight, and keep you at your healthiest. So let's find out why. The more you know about all these nutritious foods, the better equipped you'll be to "attack your fat."

Carbohydrates

Mother Nature certainly knew what she was doing when she invented carbohydrates. They're loaded with nutrients, and they're the best energy source for the human body because they provide an even, slow release of calories, keeping blood glucose levels normal. What's more, most carbohydrates provide protein, are rich in fiber, and are virtually fat free. This group includes an amazingly wide variety of foods: vegetables; fruits; legumes (beans); and grains, including breads, cereals, pasta, and foods like rice and barley. Best of all, you can eat lots of *every one* of these foods and stay slim because they're all nearly fat free.

VEGETABLES AND FRUITS

Most fresh vegetables and fruits (with the exception of olives, avocados, and coconuts) contain only a trace of fat. This makes them a great diet "bargain," provided they aren't fried or eaten with high-fat extras, such as butter, oily salad dressing, or whipped cream.

All fruits contain a good dose of fiber, particularly when eaten un-peeled, plus a wide variety of vitamins and minerals. Many are excellent sources of vitamins A and C. We need vitamin C to hold cells together and boost immune function, and researchers involved in cancer prevention recommend daily food sources of vitamin A.

According to food consumption studies, 25 percent of all Americans report that they never eat vegetables! Naturally, they should. Vegetables are loaded with vitamins, minerals, and fiber. Deep-yellow vegetables, like carrots and sweet potatoes, and dark-green leafy ones, like broccoli, are excellent sources of vitamin A. You can get your vitamin C from vegetables, too: Tomatoes, red and green peppers, Brussels sprouts, and broccoli are all good. And many vegetables, such as potatoes eaten *with* their skin, spinach, and other dark-green leafy foods, are rich in iron as well.

Crisp and crunchy raw fruits and vegetables give you lots to chew on, and they're loaded with fiber, which helps to make you feel fuller. For

FRUIT SOURCES OF TWO IMPORTANT VITAMINS

Vitamin C	Vitamin A
Orange	Mango
Grapefruit	Apricot
Tangerine	Peach
Strawberries	Nectarine
Cantaloupe	Cantaloupe
Papaya	Papaya
Watermelon	Watermelon
Persimmon	Persimmon
Pineapple, fresh	Grapefruit, pink
Guava	

all of these reasons, salads and fresh fruit make truly satisfying between-meal snacks or additions to a meal.

BREADS, CEREALS, PASTA, AND GRAINS

These starchy foods provide tremendous eating satisfaction, as well as vitamins, minerals, fiber, and virtually no fat. You just have to be careful not to sabotage them by smothering them in butter or drowning them in rich sauces.

You can eat these foods in their original grain state—like steamed brown or white rice, or cooked barley—or in prepared foods, like breads, pasta, and cereals. Remember, though, that whole-grain foods always deliver more fiber and other nutrients than those that are more processed. So try to go for whole-wheat or whole-grain bread rather than soft white bread, whole-wheat pasta as a change from the "regular" kind, and whole-grain cereals.

Most breads and pasta, unless they're made with a lot of egg (like egg noodles are) or added fats (like banana bread and croissants are), contain only one or, at most, two grams of fat per serving. The same is true for plain grains like rice, bulgur (cracked wheat), and kasha (buckwheat groats), so you can enjoy all of these delicious foods without worrying about tracking the fat. They're "free" foods.

Most ready-to-eat breakfast cereals, like wheat flakes, shredded wheat, puffed rice, corn flakes, bran, and even sweetened cereals, average about one gram of fat in an ounce. (But in specialty cereals like granola the fat count can go up: Some of these "gourmet" cereals can have four times as much fat as plain cereals.) Most cooked cereals, like corn grits, hot wheat cereal, and farina, have only a trace of fat in a serving, although oatmeal has a little more—about two grams in a serving. The real bonus that many cereals offer is soluble fiber like oat or rice bran, but we'll get to that in a minute.

WILL SUGARED CEREALS MAKE YOU FAT?

You may be surprised to learn that our answer is "No, sugared cereals *won't* make you fat." Not the ones without fat, that is. Remember, it's the *fat* in sweet things like pastries, candy bars, ice cream, and some granola cereals that will do your figure in—not the sugar.

In fact, it's time to think a little differently about sugar. While claims have been made that eating too much sugar increases the risk of obesity, diabetes, and dental cavities, research has proven that the only health problem that can be directly linked to sugar is tooth decay.

Many people enjoy sugar, and there's no reason why you shouldn't enjoy some, too. But don't go overboard; too much sugar can fill you up and crowd out the more nutritious foods in your diet. If you're craving something sweet, try some delicious fresh fruit. It's sweet and juicy, and goes wonderfully with your breakfast cereal. Or if you really need to satisfy a "sweet tooth," pick a fat-free or low-fat sugared cereal for breakfast.

Some prepared cereals contain a lot of added sugar; others have very little. But the amount of sugar in the cereal you eat really doesn't matter because it's fat that makes you fat, not sugar. The amount of sugar you get in one serving of any breakfast cereal just isn't enough to affect your weight loss. It's far more important to look for a cereal that's low in fat and high in fiber. As long as you follow those guidelines, if the cereal has some added sugar, too, enjoy it!

LEGUMES

Legumes—beans and peas, that is—come in a colorful array of shapes and sizes. You're no doubt familiar with the popular ones, like kidney beans and chick-peas (garbanzo beans), but there are literally dozens more and they all make great additions to your Fat Attack Plan.

Legumes are fat free and are packed with vitamins and minerals (like iron). They're high in fiber—the soluble kind, which helps bring your cholesterol down—and are a great appetite-satisfier. You can add them to hot meals and cold meals, to salads, soups, and stews. They're choles-terol free and very economical.

And on top of all that, you can almost consider these humble little foods the "ultimate carbs" because in addition to having all the nutri-tional virtues of their cousins—fruits and vegetables—legumes offer something more: quite a bit of protein. They're the perfect nonfat, no-cholesterol alternative to meat, cheese, and other fatty protein sources.

When you're working legumes into your eating plan, don't stop with kidney beans and garbanzos. Try lima beans, white beans, and black-eyed peas, as well as pink beans, black beans, yellow-eyed peas, and pinto beans. They're all great.

Fiber

Where weight loss and your overall health are concerned, all the carbo-hydrate foods mentioned above offer one outstanding benefit: fiber. It's naturally present in all fruits, vegetables, grains, and legumes, and the less processed the food, the more fiber you'll get.

Fiber is the substance that makes up the cell walls in plants; you can even think of it as the skeleton of plants. When you eat an unpeeled apple, you get the most fiber. When you peel the apple to make apple-sauce, the amount of fiber is reduced a great deal. If the apple is pressed to make juice or cider, very little fiber remains.

FIBER FOR WEIGHT LOSS

One of the reasons why high-carbohydrate foods are so terrific for dieters is that nature usually packages fiber in with the carbohydrates. High-fiber foods are usually very low in fat, and they're bulkier than foods without fiber. Fiber-rich foods take longer to chew. And they fill the stomach without adding any calories because fiber cannot be di-gested—it passes through the intestines without being absorbed.

Another plus is that, to some extent, fiber interferes with the absorp-tion of fat. The fat is attracted to the fiber, forming a combination that cannot be broken down; it then passes out of the digestive tract, unavail-able to the body. Fat that's not absorbed cannot make you fat because it never really enters the body.

FIBER FOR YOUR HEALTH

Fiber is an important part of the Fat Attack Plan, but weight loss isn't the only reason. Americans are being advised to eat twenty-five to forty grams of fiber a day, double the amount they usually eat. Why?

Some of the health benefits of fiber have been known for a long time. Roughage, another name for fiber, is an old remedy for constipation. More recently, however, it was discovered that in areas of the world where more fiber is eaten, digestive disorders (including constipation), diabetes, heart disease, and certain forms of cancer are much less common. But we've also learned that different kinds of fiber help prevent different kinds of illnesses.

There are actually two types of fiber: soluble and insoluble. As their names suggest, soluble fiber dissolves in water, but insoluble doesn't. Most plant foods contain both kinds of fiber, but they usually have more of one type than the other. Both soluble and insoluble fiber fill you up, but each one has specific health benefits.

SOLUBLE FIBER

Soluble fiber, the kind that will dissolve, helps you feel full and also helps lower your cholesterol and your blood sugar. Soluble fiber is believed to lower cholesterol by linking up with bile acids, which are made from cholesterol stored in the liver, and escorting them out of the body. But the bile-acid supply must be replenished, and this calls for more cholesterol, thus lowering the cholesterol circulating in the blood. And soluble fiber also slows down the body's absorption of carbohydrates, thus preventing dramatic highs and lows in blood sugar.

The best food sources of soluble fiber are apples, barley, beans, carrots, grapefruit, oats, oranges, peas, rice bran, and strawberries.

The breakfast cereals you'll eat on the Fat Attack Plan are rich suppliers of soluble fiber, which will help to lower your cholesterol. You'll be selecting from a wide variety of cereals that contain large amounts of oat and rice bran, two very effective cholesterol-lowering agents. University of Maryland researchers have found, in fact, that the soluble fiber in oat bran is just as effective in lowering cholesterol—and far less expensive —than some of the commonly used cholesterol-lowering drugs.

INSOLUBLE FIBER

Insoluble fiber, which won't dissolve, comes from the outer, hard shell of grains, and some is also found in most fruits and vegetables. It will help you feel full and has the added benefit of helping to regulate your bowels by bulking up stools. Insoluble fiber is also believed to help prevent certain forms of cancer, most notably colon/rectal cancer.

This is the kind of fiber you probably know of as the wheat bran in bran muffins and raisin bran cereal. Other excellent sources of insoluble fiber are celery, corn bran, green beans, green leafy vegetables, potato skins, and whole grains.

Protein

Protein is an important part of a balanced diet. A crucial component of every cell in our body, it's needed for tissue building and repair, and many vital bodily functions simply couldn't carry on without it.

The problem is that many Americans eat more protein than they need. Extra protein really doesn't help the body; in fact, excess protein, more than is needed to repair the body, is simply broken down. Part is used for calories and part is eliminated from the body.

Also, a lot of otherwise healthy protein sources are high in fat. Remember that there's fat hidden in the flesh of meat, chicken, and even fish— fat that can't be cut off before you eat it. As a general rule where fat content is concerned, vegetable sources of protein, like legumes, are the lowest in fat, followed by low-fat dairy foods, fish, poultry (without skin), and lean red meat, in that order.

CALCIUM

In addition to providing protein, dairy products also offer a good supply of calcium, an essential mineral. We all know that calcium is important for our bones and teeth and that well calcified bones are more resistant to adult bone thinning (osteoporosis). But according to some researchers, calcium is also an important factor in the regulation of blood pressure, possibly more important than sodium.

When you drink milk, or eat yogurt, cottage cheese, or hard cheeses, you get the same amount of calcium whether you choose the regular, reduced-fat, low-fat, or nonfat versions. So do yourself a favor and choose the dairy foods with the lowest amount of fat whenever you can. Your bones won't know the difference, but the rest of you will!

Thin Habits

As you progress through the Super Start and Getting Ahead phases of the Fat Attack Plan, you'll be learning "Thin Habits." By incorporating them into the way you eat, you'll acquire the tools you'll need, whether you're trying to lose weight or keep it off, when you're "In Control." These tips for healthier eating will help you lose weight, lower your cholesterol, improve your overall health, and even enjoy your food more.

EAT SMALL AMOUNTS FREQUENTLY

People who eat less but more often throughout the day are usually slimmer than those who eat fewer but larger meals each day. The same holds true for snackers. We all have different times during the day when we get hungry, and people who eat when they *feel* hungry rather than when the clock tells them to are thinner than those who let habit or the hour dictate mealtime. Small, frequent meals help to control diabetes and may even help to lower your cholesterol. These are among the reasons why the Fat Attack Plan offers you so many good snacks.

EAT BREAKFAST

Studies have shown that 40 percent of all adults leave the house in the morning without breakfast. Yet breakfast eaters are leaner, have lower blood pressure, eat less throughout the rest of the day, and are generally healthier than breakfast skippers. On the Fat Attack Plan you'll have satisfying, nutritious breakfasts, and eating them will *help* you lose weight or maintain your weight, whichever you're trying to do.

EAT FRUIT

Eating a piece of fresh fruit, instead of drinking fruit juice, provides more of everything: more fiber, more bulk for your stomach, more minerals, more eating time! There's more to chew, so you really feel like you've had something to eat. Fruit makes an excellent snack and a great dessert.

EAT SLOWLY

Some mornings just fly by, and before you realize it, it's lunchtime. You're in high gear from a busy morning, and you plunge into lunch at the same speed you've been working for the last few hours. Stop! Rushing through a meal this way is only going to make you feel as if you never ate at all, and you'll be far more apt to want to eat more.

Relax before you eat. Take a short walk to shift gears, or simply sit down for a few moments to catch your breath. This way you won't be eating to relieve tension and will be able to enjoy your meal. When you're eating, don't put more food into your mouth until you've swallowed the mouthful that's already there. Put your knife and fork down a couple of times during your meal. People who eat slowly eat less!

EAT IN A RELAXED ATMOSPHERE

Rushing through a meal or eating while you feel stressed can also slow down your digestion, resulting in terrible digestive turbulence: belching, heartburn, or an upset stomach. So give yourself a break if you can. Try not to eat at your desk or in the car while running errands. Mealtimes and work breaks are supposed to relieve the pressure of the day, refreshing and refueling you so that you can handle whatever else you have to take care of. Believe it or not, over fifty years ago—before life became as hurried and stressful as it is today—productivity research demonstrated that those who work without a break are actually less productive. Take some time out!

BE AWARE OF YOUR BODY'S SIGNALS

Many people don't notice how full they're getting, particularly if they're eating too quickly. You need to be better in tune with your body to keep you from eating more than you should before you've even thought about it. Stop eating for a few minutes in the middle of your meal and think about how satisfied you feel already. By the time you've finished the rest of your meal you should be feeling full.

SELECT FOODS THAT REQUIRE A LOT OF CHEWING

Crunchy low-fat foods, such as fresh vegetables, fruit, and air-popped popcorn, make great between-meal snacks—not just because they're filled with fiber, but also because you have to do a lot of chewing to get through them! The same goes for a crisp salad: It adds satisfying bulk to your meal and makes mealtime last a lot longer.

PREPARE FOOD WITHOUT ADDED FAT

On the Fat Attack Plan, you'll be learning how to cook with herbs and spices, how to marinate, how to use condiments in new ways, and how to replace your old cooking methods with new, fat-free ones. Keeping the extra fat out of your food is the best way to keep the extra fat off your body! The tips you'll learn in Super Start, Getting Ahead, and In Control are ones you'll want to stick with, not just because they'll keep your food low in fat, but also because they'll make it taste great.

CHOOSE LOW-FAT FOODS

When the choice is yours, as it will almost always be on the Fat Attack Plan, try to make the low-fat choice. For example, you'll learn the difference in fat content between regular margarine and diet margarine, between regular cream cheese and the whipped variety, and between one cut of meat and another. This way there'll be room in your "fat allowance" for a sensible portion of the special thing you'd really like to have, and your basic eating plan will be full of nutritious low-fat foods.

CHOOSE MODERATE SERVINGS OF FOOD

You'll see that there are portion sizes for each different food on the Fat Attack Plan. Don't be confused by this. Yes, there *are* lots of foods you can eat without worrying about their fat content, but it's important to eat moderate portions of all foods while you're trying to lose weight.

EAT PLAIN VEGETABLES

It probably goes without saying, but broccoli without butter or cheese sauce is less fatty than broccoli with it! Of course, you may choose to use some of your daily grams of fat to top off your vegetables; on the other hand, you can try some lemon juice or freshly ground pepper. You'll be surprised at how good these healthy foods taste without fatty adornments.

Low-Fat Living

These are the secrets of low-fat living—the things we tell our clients, the things we do ourselves—the things you can do to "eat yourself thin."

Choose the right foods: low in fat, high in fiber and other essential nutrients. Prepare them without added fat, but *with* added flavor. Eat them in the right amounts. Track the fat in fatty foods and forget about it in the others. Practice "Thin Habits."

And one more thing: enjoy! Enjoy your good food, your weight loss, your better health—*and* your longer life. How could you not, with a plan this good?

5 *Pectin Power*
A NATURAL DIET AID

Have you ever dreamed of the perfect diet aid? Something that could really help your diet along by making sure you always felt satisfied, something that might even be good for you? Something that might fall under the heading of "magic formula"?

If you have, you aren't alone. Especially if you have at least twelve to fifteen pounds to lose and start the Fat Attack Plan with Super Start, you might be feeling nervous because the menus for other weight-loss diets have left you feeling hungry. Rest assured that on Super Start you'll be free of such fears. Super Start—which, according to many of our clients, contains "an awful lot of food"—will never leave you feeling hungry and deprived. Most of you will find the menus fully satisfying. But for those of you who don't, the good news is that, in addition to all the fabulous fat-free foods we learned about in the last chapter that will help you "eat yourself thin" on the Fat Attack Plan, we've included an extra "hunger chaser" to help you chase your hunger away.

A Completely Natural Diet Aid

What is this magic "hunger chaser"? It's something that you can eat without worry, something you can buy easily at your local supermarket that's inexpensive and made of something that's very good for you. It's called pectin.

For those of you who want to use it, pectin is an important part of the Super Start phase of the Fat Attack Plan. We recommend it, and so do our clients. It's very popular with them and they've used it with great success to help them lose weight comfortably. Of course, you don't have to use it if the menus fully satisfy you. But if you want to, you simply add it to your food at lunch and dinner to help make yourself feel full longer.

If you go to the supermarket and look in the aisle where the spices and baking goods are stocked, you'll find little packages of powdered and liquid pectin. Sound familiar? This is one of the ingredients cooks use to make jam and jelly; it's the stuff that makes the fruit mixture gel so that it's thick and spreadable. Pectin is also used in the production of other foods; small amounts are used as a stabilizer (a carbohydrate that's added to thicken a product by maintaining its structure) and to improve the texture in soft cheese and yogurt.

Pectin isn't anything mysterious; it's just a food. More specifically, it's actually a fiber, one of the many different kinds of soluble fiber (that's the kind that helps lower your cholesterol). It's found in a variety of fruits and in some vegetables as well: apples, apricots, peaches, pears, plums, prunes, raisins, raspberries, raw carrots, raw onions, sweet potatoes, and beans. The peels of oranges, lemons, and grapefruit also contain a lot of this beneficial soluble fiber.

"Increased Satiety"

When researchers at the University of Southern California Medical Center were studying the effects of different kinds of fiber on digestion, they made an interesting discovery. They found that the subjects who took pectin along with their food felt full longer. In technical terms this is called "increased satiety."

The researchers concluded that it was the gelling effect of the pectin that made their subjects stay full longer. The pectin had actually made a jelly out of the food, they reasoned, making it take longer to move from their subjects' stomachs.

An Interesting Comparison

When your stomach stays fuller, you don't get hungry as soon; this is why we call pectin a "hunger chaser." And in this respect, pectin is a bit like fat: When you eat a fatty meal, it stays in your stomach longer than a meal with only a little fat, so you don't feel hungry as soon.

But this is where the resemblance ends. Fat is fat, but pectin is fiber. The big difference between fat and pectin is that when fat leaves the stomach, it's digested and absorbed as calories. But when pectin moves out of the stomach, it's not digested or absorbed; because it's fiber, it passes right out of the body in the stools. So it makes you feel full longer, but it doesn't do a thing to your figure—except improve it.

A Double Advantage

The Fat Attack Plan takes advantage of pectin's unique hunger chasing ability in the Super Start phase. By eating yogurt or cottage cheese with pectin added at lunch, and by drinking juice with added pectin at dinner, you'll feel full longer and find it easier to eat moderate amounts during the meal without feeling hungry afterward. Some of our clients report that they're full for hours after eating pectin-fortified food and never even notice if their next meal is delayed.

Pectin's other advantage, of course, is that it's a soluble fiber, the kind of fiber that has been shown to lower your blood cholesterol level as well as your blood glucose (sugar) level. A classic study showed that eating an apple a day actually reduced cholesterol in the blood by 10 percent. Apples are so rich in pectin, in fact, that no extra pectin is added when making apple jelly. And the effect of soluble fiber on diabetics has been studied by Dr. James W. Anderson of the HCF Diabetes Research Foundation, who found that when persons with diabetes eat foods high in soluble fiber, they lower their blood glucose level.

Add Pectin to Your Shopping List

When you begin your Fat Attack with Super Start, you'll get clear instructions on how and when to add pectin to your foods. But here are some other things to know about it in the meantime.

Many different companies market pectin, and you'll probably find at least two to choose from in your local grocery store or supermarket. For the Fat Attack Plan, buy any brand of powdered pectin. If you have trouble locating it in the store (the boxes *are* small), just ask the store manager for help.

These are some widely available brands:

- Sure-Jell Fruit Pectin* (General Foods)
- Sure-Jell Light Fruit Pectin* (General Foods)
- 100% Natural Fruit Pectin (Ball Corporation)
- 100% Natural Reduced-Calorie Fruit Pectin (Ball Corporation)
- Slim Set Fruit Pectin (MCP Foods, Inc.)

These products are usually made from the pectin found in apples and grapefruit, and they also contain some sugar or dextrose (a form of sugar). Some brands may also contain natural gums. But don't worry about these extra ingredients. They're just natural sugars and fibers, and they all help the pectin to gel.

There are even low-sugar or reduced-calorie varieties of pectin. The difference between these and the regular ones really isn't significant when you're on the Fat Attack Plan because they all have very little sugar

* Rabbi Y. Luban of the Kashruth Division of the Union of Orthodox Jewish Congregations of America, New York City, states that no specific certification is needed for the use of Sure-Jell.

anyway. So it doesn't matter which kind you buy, and as long as you use pectin according to the directions in "Super Start," it won't change the appearance of the food you add it to: All it will do is make it slightly thicker, and make you feel full longer.

A box of pectin is about the size of a box of dry pudding mix, and each box contains enough for three days of your Super Start eating plan. You can easily keep a box in your desk drawer, glove compartment, or purse to have handy when you need it. It needs no refrigeration or special handling once it has been opened, but to prevent spilling, it's a good idea to keep the box in a resealable plastic bag.

Any Questions?

The idea of using pectin is a new one, so we're often deluged with questions about it. Here are the things that people ask us most frequently:

Q. *Pectin has a gelling effect on the food in my stomach. But how is it different from gelatin?*
A. Pectin is a carbohydrate fiber found naturally in fruits and vegetables. Gelatin is a mixture of proteins made from animal collagen (connective tissue). We are able to digest the protein in gelatin, but we cannot digest the fiber in pectin.

Q. *Will using pectin make me uncomfortably full?*
A. No. If you use it according to our instructions, it will make you satisfied, so you won't be hungry until it's time for your next snack or meal. Remember that moderation is important for all things—including pectin. The amount we recommend on Super Start is moderate, but enough to help you.

Q. *Can I use double the amount of pectin in my yogurt or tomato juice if I want to?*
A. We don't recommend it. Instead, use pectin according to the instructions in Super Start. Remember that pectin is a food, a fiber, in fact, and like any other fiber you wouldn't want to eat too much of it.

Q. *Will it make my food taste different—sweet, maybe?*
A. Adding regular pectin will make food slightly sweeter; light pectin is a little less sweet than the regular kind. Some of our clients say they cannot tell the difference between the two. Try both and choose the one you like.

Q. *Will pectin constipate me or make me gassy?*
A. Pectin will slow down the movement of food in your stomach, but not in your digestive tract. In fact, as a fiber, pectin should help with

regularity and promote large, soft stools that are easily passed. Pectin is no more likely to cause gassiness than any other soluble fiber.

Q. *Can I use pectin as a fiber supplement every day to keep my cholesterol down, even if I'm not dieting?*

A. You could, but it isn't necessary. The Fat Attack Plan includes so many excellent food sources of fiber that you'd only need the additional pectin to aid your initial quick weight loss in Super Start. Because it helps you feel full, you eat less than you might otherwise be tempted to eat.

Q. *Have you ever tried it?*

A. Of course! We would never recommend anything to our clients that we haven't tried ourselves. Remember, pectin is a natural constituent in many of the foods you eat every day. If you're on a healthy diet, you're already eating some. And because it's a soluble fiber, little if any is absorbed by your body. Pectin will help you reduce your weight—and your health risks. Isn't it wonderful to know that there really is a natural, inexpensive diet aid that's *good* for you?

6 *Targeting Your Weight and Your Health Risks*

WHERE TO START ON THE FAT ATTACK PLAN

Most of us have a pretty good idea of how much weight we need to lose—five pounds, fifteen, maybe even thirty or more. When you can't wear most of the clothes in your closet you know it's time to lose some weight.

On the other hand, maybe you look fine the way you are. You don't need to bring your weight down, but you do need to work on your cholesterol, your triglycerides, or your blood glucose level. Or maybe your blood pressure is too high.

Whatever your health need, the Fat Attack Plan can help you. By teaching you how to remove the excess fat from your diet, it will enable you to lose weight, maintain your new weight, and improve your overall health. It takes only a few weeks on the Fat Attack Plan to lower your risk for a number of serious, possibly life-threatening diseases such as cancer, heart disease, and diabetes. And because it's a plan you can follow for life, your good health can be maintained long after you've gotten rid of those extra pounds and inches.

Which phase of the Fat Attack Plan you start with—Super Start, Getting Ahead, or In Control—depends on how much weight you need to lose, as well as the extent of your other health risks (if you have any at all). The first thing you should do is estimate a healthy and appropriate target weight for you, with the help of the guides on the next few pages. After you've done that, take the quick Health Risks Quiz that follows. We'll help you review the results of the quiz so you can put all the information together. Then look on page 53 to see just where to start your Fat Attack.

Your Target Weight

You probably already know how much you'd like to weigh. Maybe you're 142 pounds but you'd like to be 125. Or you weigh 247 but would much prefer to be 160. It will probably come as no surprise that both the average American man (who's five-foot-nine and weighs 172) and the average American woman (who's five-foot-three and weighs 143) would be a lot better off if they each lost 20 pounds.

It's important for your overall health to set a goal that's appropriate for *you*. There are a couple of different ways to do this.

ARE YOU "OVERFAT"?

First of all, how much extra fat are you carrying around? Weight is important, but it isn't everything. A pound of muscle is a lot more compact than a pound of flab! Run through these tests to see if you're "overfat."

- **Ruler Test:** Lie on your back and place a twelve-inch ruler on your stomach, pointing it from head to toe. If both ends of the ruler fail to touch your body, you're probably overfat.
- **Girth Test:** If you're wider at the waist than at the chest, you're carrying too much fat.
- **Mirror Test:** Let your eyes be the judge. If you see rolls or lumps that aren't muscle, you probably need to lose some weight.

HOW MUCH DID YOU WEIGH IN YOUR EARLY TWENTIES?

If you were a normal weight then—having completed your growth— that's probably a good weight to maintain throughout your adult life. Few of us are as trim and slim as we were at twenty-five, and the changing demands of our busy lives have a way of showing up around our hips. Most of us would love to weigh now what we weighed in our early twenties, and for most of us, that certainly isn't an impossible goal to achieve.

USE YOUR HEIGHT AND WEIGHT TO HELP YOU "GUESSTIMATE"

Another way to "guesstimate" a target weight is to use a simple formula based on your height and how much you weigh now.

WOMEN

Give yourself 100 pounds for the first 5 feet of your height and add 5 pounds for each additional inch over 5 feet (or subtract 5 pounds for each inch under 5 feet). For example, if you're 5 feet, 4 inches tall:

100 pounds (for the first 5 feet)

+ <u>20 pounds</u> (4 additional inches times 5 pounds each)

120 pounds is a desirable target weight

MEN

Give yourself 106 pounds for the first 5 feet of your height and add 6 pounds for each additional inch over 5 feet. For example, if you're 5 feet, 9 inches tall:

106 pounds (for the first 5 feet)

+ <u>54 pounds</u> (9 additional inches times 6 pounds each)

160 pounds is a desirable target weight

USING STANDARD HEIGHT AND WEIGHT TABLES TO SELECT A TARGET WEIGHT

The height and weight tables on pages 48–49 come from the Metropolitan Life Insurance Company and are based on data from insurance-policy holders. Although sometimes criticized by experts as not being the best source of weight data for all people because they are simply based on life insurance statistics, these tables are, nevertheless, widely used for estimating desirable weight. First published in 1942, the tables here were revised in 1983.

1. **The first step** in using these tables is to determine your body frame size by measuring your elbow breadth.

2. **The next step** is to locate the column for your frame size on the height and weight tables below and follow it down until it coincides with your height. The numbers you land on are the weight range for your body frame size and height. Remember that the tables assume you're wearing shoes with one-inch heels and indoor clothing. So if you're 5 feet, 3 inches barefoot, for example, you'd look under the 5-foot, 4-inch category.

Let's use Frank L. as an example. Frank has determined that his elbow breadth is 3¼ inches. This puts him in the "Large Frame" category for his height of 5 feet, 11 inches in bare feet.

Using the last column, "Large Frame," on the Height and Weight Table for Men, Frank finds the place on that column where the numbers intersect with his height. Although he's 5 feet, 11 inches, he uses 6 feet because the table assumes he's wearing shoes that add one inch to his height. Frank discovers from the table that a good target weight for his height and frame is anywhere from 164 to 188 pounds. An average weight—and thus a good target weight—for him would be about 176.

DETERMINING YOUR BODY FRAME SIZE
BY ELBOW BREADTH

To make a simple approximation of your frame size, extend your arm and bend your forearm upward at a ninety-degree angle. Keep your fingers straight and turn the inside of your wrist away from your body. Place your thumb and index finger of your other hand on the two prominent bones on *either side* of your elbow. Measure the space between your fingers against a ruler or a tape measure.* Compare your measurement with those on the appropriate table below.

These tables list the elbow measurements for medium-framed men and women of various heights. Measurements lower than those listed indicate you have a small frame; higher measurements indicate you have a large frame.

MEN

Height in 1" Heels	Elbow Breadth
5'2" – 5'3"	2½" – 2⅞"
5'4" – 5'7"	2⅝" – 2⅞"
5'8" – 5'11"	2¾" – 3"
6'0" – 6'3"	2¾" – 3⅛"
6'4"	2⅞" – 3¼"

WOMEN

Height in 1" Heels	Elbow Breadth
4'10" – 4'11"	2¼" – 2½"
5'0" – 5'3"	2¼" – 2½"
5'4" – 5'7"	2⅜" – 2⅝"
5'8" – 5'11"	2½" – 2¾"

* For the most accurate measurement, have your physician measure your elbow breadth with a caliper.

HOW MUCH DO YOU NEED TO LOSE?

Once you've made a sensible determination of what you *should* weigh, compare it with what you *do* weigh. Subtract your target weight from your current weight; the difference between these two numbers is the amount of weight you need to lose. Obviously, this is simple arithmetic.

But it's a good idea to write it down anyway. It will move you a little closer to getting started on your own personal Fat Attack Plan.

Your Current Weight _____ pounds
Less Your Target Weight _____ pounds
───────────────────────────────────
You Need to Lose _____ pounds

Targeting Your Health Risks

The following quiz will help you target your other health risks by isolating your problem areas, if any. The results of this quiz, together with the ideal weight you've just targeted, will help determine which phase of the Fat Attack Plan you should start with: Super Start, Getting Ahead, or In Control.

HEIGHT AND WEIGHT TABLES (1983)

Courtesy Metropolitan Life Insurance Company

MEN

Height	Small Frame	Medium Frame	Large Frame
5' 2"	128 – 134	131 – 141	138 – 150
5' 3"	130 – 136	133 – 143	140 – 153
5' 4"	132 – 138	135 – 145	142 – 156
5' 5"	134 – 140	137 – 148	144 – 160
5' 6"	136 – 142	139 – 151	146 – 164
5' 7"	138 – 145	142 – 154	149 – 168
5' 8"	140 – 148	145 – 157	152 – 172
5' 9"	142 – 151	148 – 160	155 – 176
5' 10"	144 – 154	151 – 163	158 – 180
5' 11"	146 – 157	154 – 166	161 – 184
6' 0"	149 – 160	157 – 170	164 – 188
6' 1"	152 – 164	160 – 174	168 – 192
6' 2"	155 – 168	164 – 178	172 – 197
6' 3"	158 – 172	167 – 182	176 – 202
6' 4"	162 – 176	171 – 187	181 – 207

(Weight in pounds according to frame; in indoor clothing weighing 5 pounds, in shoes with 1-inch heels. Weights at ages 25 to 59 are based on lowest mortality.)

WOMEN

Height	Small Frame	Medium Frame	Large Frame
4' 10"	102 – 111	109 – 121	118 – 131
4' 11"	103 – 113	111 – 123	120 – 134
5' 0"	104 – 115	113 – 126	122 – 137
5' 1"	106 – 118	115 – 129	125 – 140
5' 2"	108 – 121	118 – 132	128 – 143
5' 3"	111 – 124	121 – 135	131 – 147
5' 4"	114 – 127	124 – 138	134 – 151
5' 5"	117 – 130	127 – 141	137 – 155
5' 6"	120 – 133	130 – 144	140 – 159
5' 7"	123 – 136	133 – 147	143 – 163
5' 8"	126 – 139	136 – 150	146 – 167
5' 9"	129 – 142	139 – 153	149 – 170
5' 10"	132 – 145	142 – 156	152 – 173
5' 11"	135 – 148	145 – 159	155 – 176
6' 0"	138 – 151	148 – 162	158 – 179

(Weight in pounds according to frame; in indoor clothing weighing 3 pounds, in shoes with 1-inch heels. Weights at ages 25 to 59 are based on lowest mortality.)

HEALTH RISKS QUIZ

Circle the answer that best applies to you.

GENERAL INFORMATION

1. Age:
   A You are over 55
   B You are 55 or younger

2. Sex:
   A You are a male
   B You are a female

FAMILY HISTORY

3. One or more close blood relatives (parents, grandparents, or siblings) have had a heart attack or stroke:
   A Before age 60
   B After age 60
   C No family history of heart attack or stroke

4. One or more close blood relatives have had cancer:
   A Before age 75
   B After age 75
   C No family history of cancer
5. One or more close blood relatives have had diabetes:
   A Before age 60
   B After age 60
   C No family history of diabetes

PERSONAL HISTORY
6. You have had a heart attack or stroke:
   A Yes
7. You have diabetes:
   A Yes
8. You have had cancer:
   A Yes
9. Your total cholesterol level (in milligrams per deciliter) is:
   A 240 mg/dl or higher
   B 200 to 239 mg/dl
   C Below 200 mg/dl
10. Your LDL (low-density lipoprotein) level is:
    A 160 mg/dl or higher
    B 130 to 159 mg/dl
    C Below 130 mg/dl
11. Your HDL (high-density lipoprotein) level is:
    A Under 35 mg/dl
    B Women: 36 to 69 mg/dl
      Men: 36 to 59 mg/dl
    C Women: Over 70 mg/dl
      Men: Over 60 mg/dl
12. Your triglyceride level is:
    A Over 250 mg/dl
    B 151 to 250 mg/dl
    C 50 to 150 mg/dl
13. Your blood pressure is:
    A Higher than 160/105 (160 over 105)
    B Between 140/91 and 160/105
    C Lower than 140/90
14. Your current weight is:
    A 15 to 25 pounds over your target weight
    B 5 to 14 pounds over your target weight
    C Less than 5 pounds from your target weight

15. You smoke:

    A One or more packs a day

    B Less than one pack a day or you quit one to ten years ago

    C Never smoked or quit more than ten years ago

16. You exercise:

    A Irregularly

    B 30 minutes once or twice a week

    C 30 minutes three or more times a week

17. Stress:

    A You are easily angered, often mistrustful, impatient, or irritable

    B You are sometimes impatient, rushed, or irritable

    C You are seldom rushed or irritated; you are easygoing

RATE YOUR RISKS

Add up the number of A's, B's, and C's you circled and write them below.

A answers _____ B answers _____ C answers _____

"A" answers signal the most risk. "B" answers signal moderate risk. "C" answers indicate the least risk. If more than eight of your answers are A's, it's time to do something about your health. It's also our advice that, if over half your answers are A's or B's, you have some health risks and will benefit from the Fat Attack Plan.

While you can't change the risk you may face because of your age, sex, or family history, you can do something about the risks in questions 6 through 17.

6, 7, 8. Low-fat eating reduces the risk for both heart disease and cancer. And maintaining your target weight can help control diabetes and diminish your risk for cardiovascular illness.

9. High blood cholesterol levels have been identified as an important risk factor for heart disease. In 1987, the National Cholesterol Education Program, developed by the National Institutes of Health, issued guidelines to help Americans identify and treat high blood cholesterol. These guidelines say that adults over twenty should have a blood cholesterol of 200 milligrams per deciliter (mg/dl) or less and that cholesterol levels over 200 increase the risk for heart disease. By these standards, one in four Americans is at risk because their cholesterol is too high.

    Losing weight and lowering the total amount of fat in your diet are the two best ways to lower your total blood cholesterol.

10. Cholesterol travels through the blood as part of carriers called lipo-proteins. Low-density lipoproteins (LDLs) are the kind that contain the largest amount of cholesterol, and they're responsible for de-positing cholesterol on the artery walls. High levels of LDLs are associated with an increased risk of heart disease; the lower the LDL level the better.

    Losing weight and lowering the total amount of fat you eat are good ways to lower your LDLs.

11. High-density lipoproteins (HDLs) contain a small amount of choles-terol. They carry the cholesterol away from body cells and tissues to the liver for excretion from the body. Low levels of HDLs are there-fore associated with an increased risk of heart disease; the higher the "protective" HDL level the better.

    Losing weight, increasing exercise, and stopping smoking have been shown to increase HDLs. Moderate use of alcohol (one to two drinks a day) has also been associated with higher HDLs. This means that if you drink, you should probably limit your drinking to one or two drinks a day. Of course, if you're not a drinker, this is not a recommendation to start!

12. Almost all the fat and oil found in food and in the fat on your body are triglycerides. A high blood triglyceride level (greater than 250 milligrams) is usually an inherited disorder but can also be caused or aggravated by consuming too much caffeine or alcohol, or by abuse of vitamin A supplements.

    Losing weight, lowering the total amount of fat you eat, reducing sugars and sweet desserts, and getting more exercise have all been shown to lower blood triglycerides.

13. Blood pressure is the force of blood against the artery walls. It is measured as milliliters of mercury and reported as two numbers written like this: 120/80. The first figure (the systolic pressure) is the maximum pressure when the heart contracts. The second figure (the diastolic pressure) is the minimum pressure when the heart relaxes between beats.

    High blood pressure has been identified as an important risk factor in heart disease. Weight loss, lowering fat intake, salt restric-tion, exercise, relaxation, and avoiding smoking can all help lower high blood pressure.

14. It's important to maintain a healthy, normal weight for overall well-being. Eating less fat will help you reach the weight best for you.

15. Smoking increases your risk for many diseases, particularly cancer and heart disease. If you smoke, you are well advised to stop.

16. Exercise is a plus that will help you achieve overall good health. Be sure to get your doctor's approval before beginning an exercise program, particularly if you are at risk for heart disease.

17. The role that stress plays in overall health is controversial. In fact, recent studies show that external stress factors may not do you as much harm as being angry, hostile, or mistrustful will. But some people react to stress by eating more foods high in fat, or by overeating in general, both of which can be damaging to their health.

Where to Start Your Fat Attack

Super Start? Getting Ahead? In Control? Now that you've targeted your weight and your health risks, you can easily figure out where to start your own attack on fat.

- **If you need to lose twelve to twenty-five pounds and want to begin lowering your blood fats, blood sugar, and other health risks:**
  1. You need to begin at the beginning—with Super Start.
  2. Follow Super Start for twenty-eight days, then move on to Getting Ahead.
  3. Follow Getting Ahead for twenty-eight days. At this point you will have lost the twenty-five pounds and reached your target weight. To maintain your target weight follow In Control.
- **If your primary concern is to lower your blood fats and blood sugar, and you want to reduce your other health risks and need to lose five to fourteen pounds:**
  1. If you need to lose only a few pounds and want to lower your total cholesterol and other blood fats, skip over Super Start and move right into Getting Ahead.
  2. After four weeks, go on to In Control to maintain the healthful benefits you've achieved.
- **If you have more than twenty-five pounds to lose and need to reduce your health risks:**
  1. Don't be discouraged because you need to lose this much weight. It can be done. Begin with Super Start and follow it for twenty-eight days.
  2. Next move on to Getting Ahead, and follow it for twenty-eight days.
  3. Repeat steps 1 and 2: another twenty-eight days on Super Start, followed by another twenty-eight days on Getting Ahead.
  4. If at this point you still have some weight to lose, cycle through Super Start and Getting Ahead once again. Both of these phases of the diet are well-balanced, safe, and nutritious eating plans, and you

can keep repeating this cycle as long as you wish until you reach your target weight.

5. When you reach your target weight, move on to In Control.

6. If your current weight and your target weight are far apart, you may have to cycle through Super Start and Getting Ahead several times. But at some point you may want to give yourself a break if you feel you're getting tired of these two phases of the Fat Attack Plan. This is a good opportunity to move into In Control, a lifelong eating plan that will help you maintain your current weight loss. You may not lose much more weight while you're In Control, but you won't gain any, either. You'll be able to take a breather, get a taste of what it's like to include more fat in your daily diet, and not backslide a bit.

- **If you have no weight to lose, but want—or need—to do what you can to maintain good health and minimize your risk for major diseases:**

1. Start with In Control. If you have no weight to lose but you do want your eating habits to ensure your health in the future, In Control will do just that: help you maintain your weight; lower your cholesterol; and reduce your risk for high blood pressure, high blood cholesterol, high blood triglycerides, coronary heart disease, diabetes, cancer, osteoarthritis, gallstones, gout, and digestive upsets. At the same time you'll be In Control of what you eat, when you eat, and how much you eat.

YOU'RE ON YOUR WAY...

... to the best eating plan you've ever tried! Supported by research and shown to succeed with people like you, it's delicious and easy to follow. The Fat Attack Plan will work for you, no matter what your weight-loss or health-improvement goal. You know your target weight, and you know what your health risks are. You know where to start. So do it. Attack your fat—now!

7 *Super Start*
FAT ATTACK PLAN PHASE ONE

So, you're beginning your Fat Attack with Super Start. Congratulations! Super Start will help you achieve a quick and substantial weight loss and make you feel healthier in a short period of time—just twenty-eight days.

During that time, the preplanned Super Start menus will guide you into making low-fat eating choices. No decisions for you to make and no menu planning for you to do—unless, of course, you want to personalize your Super Start by switching meals from day to day or just repeating your favorite ones.

Whether you follow the preplanned Super Start menus or "customize" them, you'll be eating low-fat protein foods and lots of fruits, vegetables, cereals, breads, and whole grains. (Once you take a lot of the fat out of your food, you can actually eat a lot more.) And you'll be eating often—at least five times a day. But don't let that fool you. Eating small amounts, frequently, is only one of the many "Thin Habits" that you'll be learning and practicing as you progress through your Fat Attack.

The trick is to eat the right amounts of the right foods, and that you will certainly do on all the phases of the Fat Attack Plan. And even though you'll be reducing the fat in your diet, on every phase of the Fat Attack Plan—even Super Start, the most fat-restricted phase—you'll get more than enough fat to meet your body's needs. You'll get lots of fiber-rich carbohydrates to keep you satisfied at mealtimes and in between—and on Super Start you'll even have the benefit of pectin-fortified foods at lunch and dinner to help chase your hunger away.

28 Days to Success

The Super Start phase is twenty-eight days long—just the right amount of time to lose a noticeable amount of weight and start getting healthier, too. Every one of these days is packed full of good eating, and with each day that passes you'll be closer to your goal of weight loss and better health. In no time you'll be moving right into a new phase—either Getting Ahead or In Control.

A great way to record your progress and to psyche yourself into completing the first phase of your Fat Attack is to mark off each Super Start day on a calendar. If you start on a Monday, mark it as "Day 1." Tuesday becomes "Day 2," Wednesday "Day 3," and so on for each day you follow the Super Start plan. Or you can make up a calendar list like this one and cross off the days as you complete them. Twenty-eight days can go pretty fast when you're eating this well!

28 DAYS TO SUCCESS

Day 1	Day 8	Day 15	Day 22
Day 2	Day 9	Day 16	Day 23
Day 3	Day 10	Day 17	Day 24
Day 4	Day 11	Day 18	Day 25
Day 5	Day 12	Day 19	Day 26
Day 6	Day 13	Day 20	Day 27
Day 7	Day 14	Day 21	Day 28

SPECIAL OCCASIONS

But life doesn't stop just because you've changed your way of eating, and during the twenty-eight days you're on Super Start something may come up that makes it difficult to follow your preplanned menu. Maybe your neighbors invite you to a barbecue, or your best friend is throwing the most lavish wedding you'll ever attend. Or perhaps your company is having its holiday party.

Don't worry. Go ahead and enjoy an event like these once or twice during the time you're on Super Start, *but don't mark that day on your calendar*. All is not lost, and one day will not sabotage the success you've achieved so far; you've simply done what thin people do all the time. You can celebrate and eat a little extra *one day,* but then be sure to go back to making good food choices the next day and the next as well.

What you'll learn as you progress through the Fat Attack Plan is that everything you want to eat and every eating event you can imagine can be worked into a lifetime of healthy eating. An occasional hot fudge sundae, celebration meal, or midnight raid on the refrigerator will not be the downfall of all the good effort you've made so far. You just balance those occasions by making good food choices *most* of the time.

If you've followed all this advice, by the end of twenty-eight days on

Super Start you'll have lost twelve to fifteen pounds! And you'll be on your way to reducing your cholesterol, triglycerides, blood glucose, and blood pressure—a *very* successful twenty-eight days.

Super Start Thin Habits

In chapter 4 we taught you how to "eat yourself thin" and divulged a lot of the secrets of low-fat living. We also encouraged you to start getting into some new "Thin Habits." Now it's time to start putting a lot of those new habits into practice.

Thin Habits will help you lose weight *and* maintain your weight loss, by giving you the ammunition you need to get those extra pounds off and keep them off. In Super Start you'll develop Thin Habits that focus on what you eat and how you eat. Then you'll take these Thin Habits right into Getting Ahead, where you'll learn new ones that focus on selecting and eating low-fat foods. Make them habits you keep! *All* of them will serve you well when you're In Control, following the Fat Attack Plan for a lifetime of healthy eating and weight maintenance.

SUPER START THIN HABITS

In Super Start, these Thin Habits will help get you on your way to weight loss and good health:

- Eat breakfast
- Eat fruit instead of drinking juice
- Eat small amounts frequently
- Eat slowly
- Eat in a relaxed atmosphere
- Select foods that require a lot of chewing
- Be aware of your body's signals
- Prepare food without added fat

Using Pectin

In Super Start you'll be adding pectin to your food at lunch and dinner if you find your meals aren't fully satisfying and you'd like to feel fuller. (If you want all the details on this safe, completely natural "hunger chaser," go back to chapter 5 for a review.) Our clients have used pectin with overwhelming success, both because they like knowing there's a safe diet aid available if they need one and because they've found it really works.

Because pectin-fortified foods don't move out of your stomach as quickly as foods without it, we recommend it as a great way to make the satisfied feeling you get after each meal last longer. Remember that pectin is a natural soluble fiber, the kind that helps lower your cholesterol and your blood glucose (sugar) as well.

The use of pectin is optional on the Fat Attack Plan, but if you want, you'll be adding it to your yogurt or cottage cheese at lunchtime and to your tomato or other juice at dinner. If you think the menus won't be satisfying, it's worth giving it a try. It has helped a lot of other people and we think you'll be delightfully surprised at how much it can help you, too.

Using the Super Start Menus

You'll find that the Super Start menus are more structured than the menus on the other phases of the Fat Attack Plan. But that's to your benefit: We've created all these menus very carefully, to ensure delicious eating and quick weight loss with great nutrition. Yet the Super Start menus have lots of room for flexibility and your own creative choices. You can easily design meals that are more pleasing to you than the ones we suggest, if that's what you'd like to do. We want it to be easy and enjoyable for you to start your Fat Attack.

On pages 78–133 you'll find twenty-eight Super Start menus. Although these are structured menus, you'll notice that some food selections are up to you. On pages 135–41 you'll find all the food lists from which you'll be choosing things like the yogurt, cereal, or crackers you'd like to have. And if you'd like, you can personalize your Super Start menus even further by picking foods or whole meals you like from other days. Whichever way you decide to do it—follow the preplanned menus exactly or change some of the meals around—the Super Start phase will get your weight-loss diet up and running in record time.

The general rule is to use one menu each day for the next twenty-eight days. Each menu has a preplanned breakfast, lunch, dinner, P.M. Snack, and "Anytime Snack." You can begin with Day 1 and continue right through to Day 28, or you can look through the twenty-eight menus, pick the days you like best, and enjoy them in any sequence that appeals to you.

But you must do two very important—and very easy—things: First, eat! *One* breakfast, *one* lunch, *one* dinner, *one* Anytime Snack and *one* P.M. Snack each day. (Of course, on some days you may be less hungry. If that's the case, make your portions smaller, but don't skip any of your meals.) Second, follow Super Start for a full twenty-eight days, marking each of those days on your calendar.

Each day's menu in Super Start is a balanced, nutritious, low-fat eating plan for one day. If you find seven menus that you like, feel free to repeat them over and over again. *You'll achieve the same weight loss and the same positive health benefits, regardless of whether you use all twenty-eight menus or select a group that you repeat during the twenty-eight days.* If you don't use the menus for Day 1 through Day 28 consecutively, you'll find the "28 Days to Success" calendar an even greater help in keeping track of your Super Start days.

PERSONALIZING THE MENUS

Switching days around and concentrating on a few favorite days aren't the only ways to customize your Fat Attack. Another way is to switch meals between days, or even substitute foods in your meals. For example, if you like all the choices on the menu for Day 3, but you'd prefer to eat the breakfast planned for Day 4, you can easily make that switch. All the breakfasts are equal. All the lunches are equal. The same goes for all the dinners and snacks. You can mix and match as you wish.

If you want to, you can personalize a day of Super Start by eating the breakfast from Day 2, the lunch from Day 6, and the dinner from Day 28. Combining these three meals into one day along with the two snacks from Day 17 would be nutritionally equivalent to any preplanned Super Start day. Although we've done a lot of the work for you, *you* can design your own eating plan if you want to, since the possibilities for new combinations are so extensive.

THE ONE RULE YOU CANNOT BREAK

Remember that even with all this flexibility, there's one rule that can never be broken: *One* breakfast, *one* lunch, *one* dinner, *one* Anytime Snack and *one* P.M. snack *each day.*

We're happy to offer you popcorn and wine as snacks, but you can't live on them alone! Neither, for example, can you have two dinners in one day. But you can switch dinner and lunch if you want to; in fact, our clients with frequent business lunch obligations often do just that. It's just one of the many ways you can make this *your* Fat Attack.

Now let's get a taste of all the fabulous things you'll be eating on Super Start.

Breakfast

Super Start Thin Habit 1: **Eat breakfast**. Many, many people skip breakfast. They shouldn't! Unless you've been eating in your sleep, by breakfast time it will have been several hours since your last meal, and you'll need to get yourself "revved up" with a healthy breakfast if you're going to get the most out of your morning.

A LOW-FAT, HIGH-FIBER CEREAL

Each Super Start breakfast includes a serving of cereal, fruit, and milk, plus a beverage. Choose the cereal you want from the list of Cereal Choices on pages 136–37; believe it or not, there are more than fifty to choose from! All these cereals are low in fat and contain a good amount of soluble fiber—the kind that lowers your cholesterol—in the form of oats, oatmeal, or oat bran.

Each morning, have a one-ounce serving of cereal. The label on the cereal box will tell you how much there is in a one-ounce serving of that particular cereal; the serving size will be clearly stated at the top of the nutrition label. Don't assume that all cereals have about the same amount in a one-ounce serving; they can vary quite a bit, anywhere from one-fourth cup to more than a cup for an ounce.

You can eat the same cereal every morning or vary your choices. If the cereal you like isn't on the list of Cereal Choices, you may still be able to eat it during Super Start. Just check the nutrition label on the side panel of the box to see how much fat it has, and the ingredients listing to see if it contains fiber. These are the two things you need to check to see if your choice of cereal fits into Super Start. A good choice has two grams of fat or less in a one-ounce serving and contains oats, oatmeal, or oat bran.

And don't worry about the sugar content. It's fat that makes you fat, not sugar! As we learned in chapter 4, the only health problems that can be directly affected by sugar are diabetes and tooth decay. It's far more important to focus on how much fiber and fat a cereal has in it than to worry about how much sugar it contains. When you're on a low-fat eating plan like the Fat Attack Plan, the sugar in your breakfast cereal just doesn't affect your weight loss that much one way or the other.

DON'T DRINK YOUR FRUIT!

Super Start Thin Habit 2: **Eat fruit instead of drinking juice**. Each Super Start breakfast has fruit to eat rather than fruit juice to drink. Now, there's nothing wrong with fruit juice, but eating a piece of whole fresh fruit takes more time, gives you the satisfaction of chewing, and best of all adds more fiber. You can use your fruit to top your cereal, or you can eat it separately.

Remember that you can personalize. If you don't like the specific fruit planned for that day, you can substitute the fruit from any other Super Start breakfast. If you pick an alternate choice, just be sure to stick with the serving size on the list.

HAVE LOTS OF FREE DRINKS

You can choose coffee, tea, or a Free Drink with your Super Start breakfast. Free Drinks, which are listed on page 140, are beverages you can choose to have with meals or as a refreshing drink anytime during the day. Because they're "free," you can have as much of these beverages as you want. In fact, with the exception of coffee and tea, the more the better: Not only will they help you feel satisfied all day, but appreciable amounts of liquid are important for the healthy functioning of your body. Nutrition experts recommend six to eight cups of liquid daily. The Super Start menus already contain six each day; add any other Free Drinks you wish to bring this up to eight or more.

Where caffeine is concerned, be careful in your choice of beverages. Regular tea, decaffeinated coffee, and regular coffee are not Free Drinks. For one thing, research has shown that too much *coffee*—whether regular or decaf—can raise your cholesterol. All the answers are not yet in, but research shows that people who drink more than five cups of coffee per day have higher cholesterol levels. And we all know that too much caffeine (whether it comes from coffee or tea) can make you irritable and jittery. Not everyone reacts to caffeine the same way; some people are far more sensitive to its ability to act as an "upper." Two to three cups of any type of coffee or regular tea, spaced throughout the day, are fine, provided that isn't too much caffeine for you. But more than that isn't really a healthy choice.

Anytime Snack

Super Start Thin Habit 3: **Eat small amounts frequently**. Most people enjoy a midmorning snack, and depending on your breakfast and lunch schedules midmorning may be a good time of day for you to have your Anytime Snack. On the other hand, many dieters we've counseled prefer something to snack on a couple of hours after lunch. If that's your choice, save your Anytime Snack for midafternoon or for a nice break at the end of your workday. You don't even have to eat the entire Anytime Snack at one sitting—you can portion it out through the day.

Remember that snackers are leaner than non-snackers. They're usually the people who eat when they feel hungry rather than just according to what time it is. Don't worry about eating often, as long as you eat the right foods in the right amounts. Small, frequent meals are fine and will help you stick to your Fat Attack Plan.

A BAGEL A DAY—IF THAT'S WHAT YOU WANT

The Anytime Snack gives you a choice of a bagel, an English muffin, a hard roll, or two slices of most kinds of bread. Many of our clients are delighted to be able to eat a bagel every day and still lose weight. Of course, if you can't stand the idea of bagels or don't like the preplanned snack for that day, just choose another Anytime Snack—any one you like better. Remember that all the meals and snacks on the Fat Attack Plan offer lots of flexibility. If you have an English muffin you'll no doubt want it toasted, and you can certainly toast your bread or bagel, too. And if you'd like, you can enjoy your snack topped off with any type of diet jam or jelly.

Lunch

By lunchtime many of us are caught up in the pressures of a busy morning at the office or with our children, so it's easy to consider lunch just as something to fill our stomach in between demands on our time. This is the perfect opportunity to practice Super Start Thin Habits 4 and 5: **Eat slowly. Eat in a relaxed atmosphere.**

Rushing through a meal you don't even realize you're eating won't do your productivity level, your patience with your family, *or* your diet any good. What's worse, you'll miss an opportunity to enjoy a good-tasting meal like your Super Start lunch.

YOGURT

Each Super Start lunch includes a Yogurt Choice (mixed with pectin, or without if you prefer), a Lunch Cracker Choice, a Free Salad, and a Free Drink. This is really a great lunch. The salad gives you lots of chewing satisfaction, the crackers provide a nice starch accompaniment, and the yogurt is cool and creamy.

Choose the yogurt you want from the list of Yogurt Choices on pages 137–39. With more than seventy yogurts to choose from, the Super Start Yogurt Choices list is bound to offer something for almost everyone! You can eat the same yogurt every day or vary your choices.

Even if the yogurt you like isn't on the list, you may still be able to enjoy it on Super Start. But be careful. All the yogurts on the Yogurt Choices list have two grams of fat or less per serving, but *not* every brand and flavor of yogurt is low enough in fat to be included on the Yogurt Choices list. Check the nutrition panel on the yogurt container to see if it qualifies as a Super Start yogurt. A good choice has two grams of fat or less per container, which is usually an eight-ounce (one-cup) serving.

STIR IN THE PECTIN

Right before you eat your yogurt, stir in one tablespoon of powdered pectin. (It's important to wait until you're ready to eat to do this; otherwise your yogurt might separate, or get a little rubbery because it's had time to really gel.) Adding pectin to your yogurt will help you feel satisfied long after your Super Start lunch is over. Later in the day you may not even realize when it's time for your snack or dinner!

We feel that yogurt is the best choice for lunch, and our Super Start clients overwhelmingly select yogurt as their favorite lunch choice. It's available in so many flavors that it can satisfy just about everyone's preference, and it's also smooth, tasty, and nutritious. Americans love yogurt; in fact, yogurt consumption has increased over 100 percent in the last couple of years. It's one food that's gaining in popularity that's actually *good* for us.

Another plus is that a container of yogurt is an excellent source of calcium, providing 30 to 50 percent of your daily need in one serving. You'll get the rest of your daily calcium requirement from the skim milk and leafy green vegetables on the menus. Super Start menus make sure you're not shortchanged on this or any other important minerals while you're losing weight.

(One more thing: Be sure to eat your yogurt even if you don't add pectin to it. It's an important part of your balanced diet during Super Start.)

ANOTHER SUPER START LUNCH OPTION

Some people prefer to vary their lunch menu a little. If that's what you'd like, you may have one cup of any *low-fat* cottage cheese—even the kind with vegetables or fruit in it—instead of yogurt. (Stir your pectin into the cottage cheese the same way you'd do for yogurt, right before you eat it.) Cottage cheese is similar in nutritional value to yogurt, but it has a lot less calcium. Because one cup provides only 15 percent of your daily calcium requirement, it's not a good idea to switch cottage cheese for yogurt more than twice a week. (And be sure to have your yogurt or cottage cheese, even if you're not adding pectin.)

Something that makes a nice change—and a nice combination—is to have a half-cup of cottage cheese and a half-cup of yogurt. (Just be sure to split your pectin, if you're using it, between the two.) Having a half-cup of each is another example of how you can personalize and add some variety to your Super Start meal. You might even want to have your salad with a half-cup of cottage cheese and your crackers as your "main dish," and then enjoy a half-cup of yogurt as "dessert."

YOUR CRACKER CHOICE

Each lunch has a preplanned Cracker Choice. There are quite a few crunchy, low-fat selections to choose from on the list on page 139. If you don't like the selection on the preplanned menu for the day, just choose another cracker or any other item from the list. You can even choose unbuttered popcorn if you'd like it; it's right there on the list and it's a fun change.

FREE SALAD

Your Super Start lunch also includes a Free Salad—as much of it as you'd like. You get to invent a Free Salad every day from the *long* list of Free Salad Fixings on pages 139–40. You decide which items and how much of each to put in your salad bowl. These Salad Fixings are "free" foods because they're virtually fat free. Have as much as you want—Salad Fixings are unlimited.

One of the great things about a nice big salad is that you get to munch on it for a long, long time! Super Start Thin Habit 6: **Select foods that require a lot of chewing.** Not only will a food that requires a lot of chewing make your mealtime last longer, but these foods are often the ones that are highest in fiber and lowest in fat.

FREE DRESSING

You may enjoy your Free Salad plain or you may be happy with a dash of flavored vinegar. There are so many fragrant new vinegars on the market these days, like raspberry vinegar or those flavored with herbs, that you might want to treat yourself to a bottle or two. Or maybe you'd like a squeeze of fresh lemon or lime juice and some freshly ground pepper. Many of the suggestions on the Free Condiments list on pages 140–41 can be used to "dress" a salad, too. If you'd like a spicy tomato-based salad dressing, make up a batch of our fat-free "Zero Dressing;"

the recipe is on page 78. Zero Dressing is as fat free as its name implies, so you can use it liberally on your salad.

But if you don't feel like making your own salad dressing, or want a greater variety, check the salad dressing aisle in your supermarket for "no-oil" dressings. These are prepared dressings that contain no oil, or salad dressing mixes that are made without added oil. When you read the nutrition label on a "no-oil" salad dressing, make sure it contains no fat (0 grams). As long as it's fat free, you can use as much of this kind of dressing as you'd like to top off your Free Salad.

Now that you've enjoyed a filling, nourishing lunch, stop for a moment to think about how satisfied you are. Super Start Thin Habit 7: **Be aware of your body's signals**. Right now your body is saying, "I've been fed— thank you." Realizing that you're full and that your meal is over now will keep you from eating more than you should. And don't forget: There's a snack or another meal just a few hours away.

Dinner

Each Super Start Dinner includes tomato juice (or your choice of several other juices) mixed with pectin; a Main Dish of meat, fish, or poultry; a Side Dish; a vegetable; a Free Salad; and your choice of coffee, tea, or a Free Drink.

A BEFORE-DINNER "COCKTAIL"

Get your dinner—or even your cocktail hour—off to a Super Start with a special Fat Attack "cocktail" that packs its own healthy kind of punch: a pectin-fortified tomato juice cocktail complete with a "swizzle stick" of celery or cucumber.

Choose tomato juice or any of the other Dinner Juice Substitutes from the list on page 139. Then add one tablespoon of powdered pectin to the juice. Pour the pectin in slowly, stirring to combine it with the juice. The pectin will help you feel full so that you can enjoy your dinner without overeating. It will also prevent you from getting an attack of the "after-dinner munchies," because you'll feel satisfied longer.

For a change from tomato juice, try vegetable, Beefamato, Clamato, or any of the others on the Dinner Juice Substitutes List. Any of these substitutes is fine, but they are the only juice varieties you can use. The physical and chemical properties of tomato juice (or other tomato-based juices), as well as the way it's processed, make it one of the best juices for dissolving pectin.

You'll notice that grapefruit juice is the only fruit juice on the list. Orange juice and most nectars have naturally occurring acids and sometimes enzymes that break down the gelling action of pectin. Grapefruit juice does make a nice change from tomato juice, but don't forget that there are lots of things you can do with your tomato juice. Spice it up with pepper, lemon juice, Worcestershire sauce, or horseradish. Decorate it with a big leafy stalk of celery, which you can munch on as you enjoy your drink. Or check out page 98 for even more ideas on how to add zip to your Super Start "cocktail."

(Remember, these are pectin "cocktails," not alcoholic drinks. We do not recommend adding any kind of liquor to this kind of cocktail. And don't forget to have your tomato juice even if you've chosen *not* to have pectin with it.)

Your Main Dish

Each Super Start menu has a preplanned Main Dish of meat, fish, or poultry. You may, if you wish, replace the preplanned Main Dish with any other preplanned Main Dish on Super Start. Remember, though, if you select a different Main Dish, you must use the portion size indicated.

All the portion sizes on the menus are given in ounces and refer to the weight of the meat only, after cooking, minus the bone and fat. When you're at the market, select a piece of raw meat, fish, or poultry that's one ounce heavier than the suggested portion size; at that portion size you can safely assume that you'll lose about one ounce in cooking.

COOKING WITHOUT ADDED FAT

Super Start Thin Habit 8: **Prepare foods without added fat.** All Main Dish selections should be prepared with no added butter, oil, shortening, margarine, or cream.

Before you balk, let us assure you that it's a lot easier and a lot tastier (not to mention healthier) than you may think it is to cook this way. First of all, you may use a cooking spray to "grease" a pan or to lightly coat foods so they can be sautéed. But that's just the beginning. Here are more tips to help you prepare deliciously low-fat Super Start dinners.

• **Marinate**. Marinate meats, poultry, or fish in any combination of lemon juice, lime juice, flavored vinegar, or pickle juice (yes, pickle juice!). You can also have hot sauce, salsa, horseradish, ginger, garlic, or your favorite herbs and spices. For even more ideas on what to marinate in, see the Free Condiments list on pages 140–41.

Spread the top of the food you're preparing with a mixture of mustard, salsa, and/or diet jelly, plus your favorite seasonings. Fish usually needs more delicate treatment: Drizzle it with lemon or lime juice, then sprinkle on your favorite herbs. You'll find more suggestions for marinades in the Super Start menu section.

- **Use herbs and spices.** This is a simple and easy way to add flavor and elegance to the most simple dish. If you're unsure of how to do this, begin with the classic combinations—tomatoes with basil, parsley with fish, rosemary with chicken—and experiment with other combinations as your confidence grows. The Flavorings chart that follows will provide you with many more ideas to try. And the best part is that you can use herbs and spices without worry, because they're fat free.

SOME FAVORITE FLAVORINGS

Herbs are available both fresh and dried. Many cooks feel that fresh herbs impart the best flavor, but good dried herbs work wonderfully, too. Just remember that *3 teaspoons of a fresh herb are equal to 1 teaspoon of the same herb dried.*

Most recipes call for ground spices, although many spices are available in whole dry form. Remember that *1½ teaspoons of a whole dry spice are equal to ½ teaspoon of that same spice ground.*

Herb or Spice	Popular Use
Allspice	Fish, shellfish, sweet potatoes
Anise	Fish, shellfish
Basil	Fish, poultry, all meats, green salads, tomatoes, most vegetables
Bay leaf	Fish, all meats (especially lamb)
Borage	Fish, shellfish, salads, green leafy vegetables
Burnet	Salads
Capers	Fish, salads, tomatoes, eggplant
Camomile	Poached meat
Caraway	All meats, cabbage, turnips
Cardamom	Sweet potatoes
Cayenne	"Hot," on any food
Celery seed	Cabbage, potatoes
Chervil	Fish, shellfish, green salads
Chives	Fish, baked potatoes, salads
Cilantro	Ground meat, beans, stir-fried dishes, salads, Mexican foods
Cinnamon	Pork, fruits
Clove	Pork

Herb or Spice	Popular Use
Cumin	Ground meat, cabbage
Dill	Fish, shellfish, all meats, cucumbers, salads
Fennel	Chicken, fish, shellfish
Filé powder	Adds Creole flavor to foods
Ginger	Fish, shellfish, poultry, all meats, stir-fried dishes
Horseradish	Fish, shellfish, all meats
Hyssop	Vegetables, salads
Lemon balm	Fruits
Lemon verbena	Fruits
Mace	Fish
Marjoram	Lamb, poultry, salads, green vegetables
Mint	Lamb, beans, peas, fruits
Mustard	Beets; adds zest to most foods
Nutmeg	Vegetables
Oregano	Fish, ground meat, tomatoes
Paprika	Fish, potatoes, salads
Parsley	Fish, all meats, poultry, salad, vegetables
Pepper, black (zesty) **and** Pepper, white (mild)	Fish, shellfish, all meats, poultry, salad, vegetables, pasta, rice
Rosemary	Beef, lamb, pork, chicken, vegetables
Saffron	Fish, shellfish
Sage	Fish, shellfish, pork, veal
Savory	Fish, shellfish, ground meat, poultry, lentils, beans, cabbage, peas, tomatoes
Sorrel	Salads
Sweet cicely	Salads, vegetables
Tarragon	All meats, poultry, tomatoes, salads
Thyme	Clams, fish, all meats, poultry, tomatoes
Turmeric	Fish, shellfish, chicken, noodles, pasta, rice

Herb and Spice Blends	Popular Use
Apple pie spice	All fruits
Barbecue spice	Broiled meats, ground meat, chicken, potatoes, salads
Bouquet garni	Poached foods

Chiffonade of fresh herbs	Poached foods
Chili powder	Ground meat, salads
Chinese five-spice powder	All meats, poultry, stir-fried dishes
Crab boil	Fish, shellfish, poultry, all meats, beans, rice, vegetables
Curry powder	Fish, shellfish, poultry, all meats, beans, rice, vegetables
Fines herbes	Salads
Pickling spice	Marinated vegetables
Pizza seasoning	Chicken, ground meat, tomato sauce
Poultry seasoning	Fish, shellfish, ground meat, poultry
Pumpkin pie spice	Winter squash

- **Cook it correctly.** The best cooking methods for preparing Super Start dinner selections are dry broiling, grilling, roasting, poaching, and steaming. A basic cookbook will give you standard cooking times for fish, meat, and poultry. Cook until done, but remember that without added fat, only the natural juices will keep your foods moist. This works wonderfully as long as you don't let your dinner overcook.

- **Try poaching.** A great way to prepare moist, delicious entrées is to poach them. Fish and boneless chicken take particularly well to this classic cooking method. Place the fish or chicken in just enough simmering water to barely cover, then add lemon slices, celery leaves, whole peppercorns, and any other spices or herbs you'd like. Poach anywhere from a couple of minutes for shellfish to about twenty minutes for chicken; check your cookbook for more specific poaching times.

- **Jazz it up.** Garnish your Main Dish with any of the Free Salad Fixings on pages 139–40 or with a Free Condiment from the list on pages 140–41. You may find that in Super Start you're paying more attention to preparing and "presenting" your dinner dishes than you have in a while. That's good. Taste and nutrition are very important, but fussing over your food can be fun, too. Particularly when you're dieting, it's nice to treat yourself and your family to something that looks pretty. You deserve it!

And on the Side...

Along with your Main Dish, each Super Start menu has a preplanned serving of a Side Dish of potatoes, rice, pasta, grain, or beans. If you don't like the preplanned choice, pick an alternate from another Super Start dinner. Just be sure to use the serving size given on the list when you do this; that way you'll be sure that your substitution is an equal one.

HAVE IT HOWEVER YOU LIKE IT...

... as long as it doesn't have any added fat. You can bake or boil the potatoes; steam the rice, bulgur, or groats; and boil the pasta or beans. Just be sure to prepare your Side Dish without any added fat. There are lots of ways to do this.

If you want a change from boiled or steamed **potatoes**, mashed potatoes are another option, and you really can prepare them without fat! Steam or boil potatoes, then peel and mash them, mixing in a little skim milk. Add plain or seasoned pepper and salt, if you wish, then garnish with some butter sprinkles and chopped parsley. Butter sprinkles are a fat-free, cholesterol-free, all-natural butter substitute that you can use when you want butter flavor. If you're in a hurry, you can use instant mashed potatoes, preparing them with water and skim milk instead of whole milk, omitting the margarine or butter. Flavor them instead with butter sprinkles and the same seasonings you'd use for fresh mashed potatoes. To boost the calcium and add a richer flavor, just reverse the proportions of milk and water: Now you'll be adding more milk than water.

Sweet potatoes can be steamed, baked, or mashed. Fresh ones are delicious, but canned sweet potatoes packed in water or syrup are a good substitute. Just heat and serve however you'd like.

Pasta—and grains like rice, buckwheat groats (kasha), and bulgur (cracked wheat) can all be combined with any of the Free Salad Fixings listed on pages 139–40 and seasoned with any of the Free Condiments on the list on pages 140–41. Take a look at Days 2, 7, 9, 22, 23, and 26 for some good ideas on grains and how to prepare them. Check the Flavorings chart on pages 67–69 for inspiration on adding extra flavor to these wonderful basic foods.

For example, spray a pan with cooking spray and sauté a few chopped mushrooms and one or two chopped green onions for a few minutes, until they've softened. Then mix the vegetables into cooked rice, pasta, kasha, or bulgur and season with your favorite herbs or spices.

You can use any variety of canned or frozen **beans**. Of, if you wish, you can cook them from scratch—but this takes a long time, so we suggest you cook an entire pound at a time. Then separate them into half-cup portions and freeze them. They'll be ready, all measured out, when you need them. Small resealable plastic bags make good freezer storage containers that can go directly into the microwave for reheating.

All varieties of beans can be flavored quickly with any herb or spice. Or try chopped onions, green onions, celery, cucumbers, garlic, hot peppers, parsley, cilantro, radishes, or any of the other Free Salad Fixings listed on pages 139–40. You can add Free Condiments from pages 140–41; these are great if you want to make a cold bean salad. Or do it with flavored vinegar—just mix and chill.

You're probably wondering why **noodles** aren't included on the Side Dishes list. This is because most noodles are made with eggs and therefore contain fat. But all the other pasta choices are fat free. If you can find "no-egg" or "no-egg-yolk" noodles, though, these are fine. Use them in your Super Start dinners and enjoy!

VEGETABLES AND SALAD

Each Super Start menu includes a preplanned vegetable. You don't have to have the one on the menu, but in that case do be sure to pick one from another Super Start dinner and include it in your meal. It can be cooked or raw; that doesn't matter.

What does matter is eating the correct amount. Even though vegetables are virtually fat free, it's wise right now, while you're trying to lose weight quickly, to use a one-cup serving as the list indicates. It's important during Super Start to teach yourself to eat moderate portions. Later on in the Fat Attack Plan, vegetables will be a "free food," and you'll be able to have as much of them as you'd like.

To add a little flavor to vegetables, zest them up with a squeeze of fresh lemon juice, or try the same suggestions for cooking beans. Butter sprinkles, a fat-free butter substitute, can add the buttery flavor you love on vegetables without sabotaging your diet. Remember that you can also sauté any of the Free Salad Fixings in a skillet prepared with cooking spray and add them to your vegetable for flavor and color.

And—as if all of this weren't enough to keep you full for quite a while —you also get a big Free Salad for dinner. This is one of the best parts of the Super Start Menus. You can concoct any combination of vitamin- and fiber-filled greens and garnishes from the long list of Free Salad Fixings on pages 139–40 and munch away to your heart's content—every night!

P.M. Snack

Many travelers feel a hotel isn't a hotel if they don't get a mint on their pillow each night. Well, the Fat Attack Plan doesn't offer you a mint, but how about a piece of fruit, some popcorn, or a glass of wine instead?

It's nice to be able to end the day with a little something to sip or nibble on, and we've worked that into Super Start because we want your new eating plan to be enjoyable as well as nutritious and sound. Remember, "Eat small amounts frequently" is a Thin Habit. So enjoy your snack —it's *good* for your Fat Attack.

Each Super Start menu has a preplanned P.M. Snack. But if you don't want the preplanned one, you can substitute one from any other Super Start day. That might mean a different fruit, or four ounces of any dry or semi-dry (but not sweet) wine.

WHY WINE?

Many people enjoy a glass of wine in the evening, and since it's fat free you can continue to enjoy it—in moderation, of course. That's why we've built in one glass a day.

Wine has some special benefits. It's low in sodium, it increases mineral absorption, and it aids in the digestive process. Most wines have a beneficial effect on blood fat levels. Wine is also a tension reliever, it helps control anxiety, and it promotes longer, more restful sleep.

If you feel like munching at snack time, two cups of air-popped popcorn (without butter) and a nice Free Drink should satisfy the urge. Feel free to have your snack anytime after dinner: Use it as a dessert, as a TV snack, or as a bedtime treat.

Moving Along

With this many good things to eat, your twenty-eight days on Super Start are sure to fly by. Before you know it, you'll have lost twelve to fifteen pounds and will be healthier, too! Then it will be time to move on to Getting Ahead, the next phase of your Fat Attack. By the time you finish Getting Ahead, you'll have reached your weight-loss goal of twenty-five pounds and will have reduced your risk for many major diseases.

If twenty-five pounds was what you wanted to lose, you'll be ready to move into In Control for a lifetime of low-fat eating and good health. But if your targeted weight loss was more than twenty-five pounds, recycle back into Super Start and then through Getting Ahead one more time, or until you reach your target weight.

LEARNING AS YOU LOSE

You may wonder why we don't recommend that you just stay on Super Start until you've lost all the weight you want to. There are a couple of reasons for spending twenty-eight days with Super Start and then twenty-eight days with Getting Ahead.

First of all, it relieves you of being on a restricted eating plan for too long a stretch.

Just as important, the Fat Attack Plan is designed to teach you how to make low-fat food choices. You'll learn some of these on Super Start and even more of them on Getting Ahead, where you'll also have a chance to put them into practice. We want you to have the opportunity to practice what you've learned, and Getting Ahead provides you with that opportunity.

Alternating between these two Fat Attack phases also solves another major problem that dieters face: boredom. Many weight-loss diets just don't offer enough variety, so the dieter gets bored and goes off the diet before accomplishing his or her goal. But by cycling through one phase first and then moving on to a different phase, you get variety. And on Getting Ahead you also have the fun of making Fat Choices, a great reward for all the effort you put into Super Start.

Our clients have shown us over and over again that this works. They cycle through Super Start and Getting Ahead until they've reached their goal, and then—regardless of what phase they're in—they move right into In Control as soon as they achieve their target weight.

It's the best reward of all—a delicious eating plan that really doesn't say no to anything and a longer lifetime of good health to enjoy it in. It can be your reward, too. Start marking your "28 Days to Super Start Success" today!

Super Start
MENUS

The following twenty-eight preplanned menus are for use during Super Start. You can use one each day for the next twenty-eight days, beginning with Day 1 and going right through to Day 28. Another option is to look over the twenty-eight menus and pick the ones you like best, repeating them over and over until you've followed Super Start for twenty-eight days. The "28 Days to Success" Calendar on page 56 will help you keep track of the days if you don't use the menus for Day 1 through Day 28 in order.

You're ready to Super Start!

Super Start
MENU PATTERN

BREAKFAST
Cereal
Fruit
Skim Milk
Coffee, Tea, or Free Drink

ANYTIME SNACK
Bagel or Bread
Coffee, Tea, or Free Drink

LUNCH
Yogurt plus Pectin
Free Salad
Crackers
Free Drink

DINNER
Tomato (or Other Dinner) Juice plus Pectin
Main Dish
Side Dish
Vegetable
Free Salad
Coffee, Tea, or Free Drink

P.M. SNACK
Fruit or Wine or Popcorn

PERSONALIZING THE
Super Start
MENU PATTERN

The preplanned Super Start menus offer you many chances to choose your favorite foods throughout the day. For each underlined menu item below, refer to the food list on the page indicated to make your choice.

BREAKFAST
Cereal (pages 136–37)
Fruit
Skim Milk
Coffee, Tea, or Free Drink (page 140)

ANYTIME SNACK
Bagel or Bread
Coffee, Tea, or Free Drink (page 140)

LUNCH
Yogurt (pages 137–39) **plus** *Pectin*
Free Salad (pages 139–40)
Crackers (page 139)
Free Drink (page 140)

DINNER
Tomato (or Other Dinner) Juice (page 139) **plus** *Pectin*
Main Dish
Side Dish
Vegetable
Free Salad (pages 139–40)
Coffee, Tea, or Free Drink (page 140)

P.M. SNACK
Fruit or Wine or Popcorn

ZERO DRESSING

Makes 1½ cups

1 cup tomato juice
½ cup lemon juice
2 tablespoons chopped onion
⅛ teaspoon pepper
1 teaspoon chopped fresh parsley or ¼ teaspoon dried
1 clove garlic, minced
¼ teaspoon dry mustard
2 tablespoons chopped bell pepper (optional)

Combine all ingredients in a tightly covered container; shake to blend. Store in refrigerator.

TIP ▬▬▬▬▬▬▬▬▬▬▬▬▬▬▬▬▬▬▬▬▬▬▬▬

Skim milk is a good choice when you want less fat.

1 cup skim milk has a trace of fat
1 cup low-fat (1%) milk has 3 grams of fat
1 cup whole milk has 8 grams of fat

Super Start
MENU—DAY 1

BREAKFAST
1 Ounce Cereal Choice
1 Medium Grapefruit
1 Cup Skim Milk
Coffee, Tea, or Free Drink

ANYTIME SNACK
1 Bagel
Coffee, Tea, or Free Drink

LUNCH
*1 Container Yogurt **plus** Pectin*
*Free Salad **plus** Zero Dressing*
2 Rice Cakes
Free Drink

DINNER
*1 Cup Tomato Juice **plus** Pectin*
3 Ounces Broiled Flank Steak
1 Large Baked Potato
1 Cup Steamed Broccoli
*Free Salad **plus** Zero Dressing*
Coffee, Tea, or Free Drink

P.M. SNACK
1 Medium Pear

TIP ▬▬▬▬▬▬▬▬▬▬▬▬▬▬▬▬▬▬▬▬▬▬▬▬▬▬▬▬

It makes sense to remove the skin from chicken.

½ chicken breast, roasted, without skin has 3 grams of fat
½ chicken breast, roasted, with skin has 8 grams of fat

Eating the chicken skin almost triples the fat!

TIP ▬▬▬▬▬▬▬▬▬▬▬▬▬▬▬▬▬▬▬▬▬▬▬▬▬▬▬▬

RICE PILAF

For a nice change from plain rice: *Combine ¾ cup water and 1 teaspoon powdered chicken bouillon or ½ small chicken bouillon cube; bring to a boil and add ¼ cup enriched long-grain rice; cover, reduce heat to simmer, and cook for 10 minutes.*

Stir into the partially cooked rice 1 tablespoon chopped onion, 1 teaspoon chopped fresh parsley, and 2 tablespoons diced celery.

Cook 10 minutes longer or until all the liquid is absorbed and the rice is soft. Makes one serving.

TIP ▬▬▬▬▬▬▬▬▬▬▬▬▬▬▬▬▬▬▬▬▬▬▬▬▬▬▬▬

You might enjoy diet jam or diet jelly with your Anytime Snack bread choice. Because these are Free Sweets, you can include them in your Super Start Menu Pattern.

Super Start
MENU—DAY 2

BREAKFAST
1 Ounce Cereal Choice
1 Large Orange
1 Cup Skim Milk
Coffee, Tea, or Free Drink

ANYTIME SNACK
1 English Muffin
Coffee, Tea, or Free Drink

LUNCH
*1 Container Yogurt **plus** Pectin*
*Free Salad **plus** Zero Dressing*
3 Pieces Norwegian Crispbread
Free Drink

DINNER
*1 Cup Tomato Juice **plus** Pectin*
½ Roasted Chicken Breast (without skin)
¾ Cup Steamed Rice
1 Cup Steamed Peas
*Free Salad **plus** Zero Dressing*
Coffee, Tea, or Free Drink

P.M. SNACK
4 Ounces Dry or Semi-dry Wine

Surimi (shellfish substitute) is a widely available, less-expensive substi-tute for shellfish. It is equally low in fat.

Surimi is already cooked when you buy it. Try soaking it in cold water for 30 minutes before using to remove excess salt and freshen the taste.

Surimi can be used to make this dinner, hot or cold.

FOR A HOT SEAFOOD DINNER
Try this combo meal: *Combine ⅓ cup buckwheat groats (kasha) in ⅔ cup water; bring to a boil and cook over medium heat 10 minutes. Add 1 tablespoon sliced scallions and ½ cup mung bean sprouts and surimi. Cook 3 minutes longer.*

FOR A COLD SEAFOOD DINNER
Cook and cool groats and snow pea pods. Combine with some Zero Dressing or toss with some flavored vinegar. Prepare your Free Salad, top it off with surimi, and dress with the snow pea/groat mixture you made.

To enjoy a wide variety of breads while on Super Start, store bread in the freezer, taking out slices only as needed. Sliced bread defrosts in a few minutes, or it can be toasted or warmed in the microwave.

Super Start
MENU—DAY 3

BREAKFAST
1 Ounce Cereal Choice
1 Small Banana
1 Cup Skim Milk
Coffee, Tea, or Free Drink

ANYTIME SNACK
2 Slices Whole Wheat Toast
Coffee, Tea, or Free Drink

LUNCH
*1 Container Yogurt **plus** Pectin*
*Free Salad **plus** Zero Dressing*
2 Pieces Wasa Crispbread
Free Drink

DINNER
*1 Cup Tomato Juice **plus** Pectin*
*4 Ounces Shellfish Substitute (Surimi) **or** Crabmeat*
3/4 Cup Steamed Buckwheat Groats (Kasha)
1 Cup Steamed Snow Pea Pods
*Free Salad **plus** Zero Dressing*
Coffee, Tea, or Free Drink

P.M. SNACK
1 Medium Apple

TIP

Mash baked sweet potato with 2 teaspoons diet marmalade and sprinkle with cinnamon. Or, try sprinkling it with butter sprinkles and add a dusting of nutmeg.

TIP

Many people think of ham as a fatty, salty food. It doesn't have to be. Next time you shop, check the "deli" counter or meat case for extra-lean ham.

1 ounce lean ham has 1 gram of fat
1 ounce regular ham has 3 grams of fat—three times as much

Low-salt varieties are also available.

Stay away from minced ham, chopped ham, and canned or prepared ham salad. All are higher in fat than regular ham and much higher in fat than the extra-lean variety.

TIP

For an attractive dinner plate and a new taste treat: Spread each ham slice lightly with a tasty, pungent mustard and roll it around a few spears of asparagus before serving.

Super Start
MENU—DAY 4

BREAKFAST
1 Ounce Cereal Choice
1 Kiwi
1 Cup Skim Milk
Coffee, Tea, or Free Drink

ANYTIME SNACK
2 Slices Rye Bread
Coffee, Tea, or Free Drink

LUNCH
1 Container Yogurt **plus** *Pectin*
Free Salad **plus** *Zero Dressing*
4 Pieces Cracklebread
Free Drink

DINNER
1 Cup Tomato Juice **plus** *Pectin*
4 Ounces Baked Lean Ham
1 Medium Baked Sweet Potato
1 Cup Steamed Asparagus Spears
Free Salad **plus** *Zero Dressing*
Coffee, Tea, or Free Drink

P.M. SNACK
2 Cups Air-popped Popcorn

QUICK GAZPACHO

Makes four 1-cup servings

1 clove garlic
1 small onion, coarsely chopped (2 tablespoons)
1 large cucumber, peeled and chunked
1 green pepper, seeded and chunked
1 fresh tomato, cut in quarters
2 cups tomato juice
Juice of ½ lemon
½ teaspoon chili, or to taste

Finely process garlic and onion in a blender or food processor. Add cucumber, pepper, and tomato; pulse to chop coarsely. Add tomato juice, lemon juice, and chili; pulse to combine. Refrigerate in a tightly covered container for a few hours to blend flavors. Will keep for up to one week.

This delicious alternative to tomato juice has no fat. One cup does have 223 milligrams of sodium. For less sodium, try using low-sodium tomato juice; 1 cup has only 6 milligrams of sodium.

Be sure to add your pectin just before serving.

When buying a raw piece of meat "bone-in" such as a chop, buy one 5-ounce chop to yield a 3-ounce edible portion. Three ounces of meat remain after cooking and discarding the bone and fat from a 5-ounce chop.

Super Start
MENU—DAY 5

BREAKFAST
1 Ounce Cereal Choice
1¹/₂ Cups Strawberries
1 Cup Skim Milk
Coffee, Tea, or Free Drink

ANYTIME SNACK
1 Bagel
Coffee, Tea, or Free Drink

LUNCH
1 Container Yogurt plus Pectin
Free Salad plus Zero Dressing
2 Pieces Melba Toast
Free Drink

DINNER
1 Cup Quick Gazpacho plus Pectin
3 Ounces Broiled Veal Chop (meat only)
1 Cup Boiled Potato
1 Cup Steamed Zucchini
Free Salad plus Zero Dressing
Coffee, Tea, or Free Drink

P.M. SNACK
4 Ounces Dry or Semi-dry Wine

KIDNEY-BEAN SALAD

Mix ¾ cup cooked or canned kidney beans with 1 tablespoon no-oil salad dressing, 1 sliced scallion (white and green parts), and 2 tablespoons chopped yellow pepper. Add salt and pepper to taste and serve at room temperature.

Prick frankfurter with a fork before pan-frying in a nonstick skillet. Some fat will cook out, so you'll get less. Pat frankfurter with a napkin before eating to remove even more fat.

Chicken and turkey frankfurters have less fat than beef or pork varieties.

1 chicken frankfurter has 9 grams of fat
1 turkey frankfurter has 8 grams of fat
1 beef frankfurter has 13 grams of fat
1 beef and pork frankfurter has 17 grams of fat

Frankfurters usually contain nitrates, food additives that sometimes convert themselves into nitrosamines. This can happen before the food is even prepared, or after it has been eaten, during the digestive process. Nitrosamines have been identified as carcinogens (substances that may cause cancer).

However, the vitamin C in the tomato juice you have at dinner prevents the formation of nitrosamines. So it's good to have a vitamin C–rich food whenever you eat foods preserved with nitrates.

Super Start
MENU—DAY 6

BREAKFAST
1 Ounce Cereal Choice
½ Mango
1 Cup Skim Milk
Coffee, Tea, or Free Drink

ANYTIME SNACK
2 Slices Whole Wheat Toast
Coffee, Tea, or Free Drink

LUNCH
*1 Container Yogurt **plus** Pectin*
*Free Salad **plus** Zero Dressing*
2 Cups Air-popped Popcorn
Free Drink

DINNER
*1 Cup Tomato Juice **plus** Pectin*
*1 Chicken **or** Turkey Frankfurter*
¾ Cup Cooked Kidney Beans
1 Cup Steamed Green Beans
*Free Salad **plus** Zero Dressing*
Coffee, Tea, or Free Drink

P.M. SNACK
1 Cup Fresh Pineapple

TO FLAVOR TRICOLOR PASTA

Steam 1 cup shredded escarole and ¼ cup sliced celery. Add ½ teaspoon minced garlic and 1 tablespoon chopped fresh basil. Combine with hot pasta.

Many salad greens, especially the deep green kinds, are especially important sources of vitamins and minerals.

Escarole, Romaine and red-leaf lettuce are rich in vitamin A. In fact, a salad made with Romaine can supply as much as half your daily need. Iceberg and looseleaf lettuce are rich in vitamin K. Spinach is high in iron and other minerals. All salad greens are good sources of potassium.

And remember to always eat your parsley garnish—a great source of vitamin A, vitamin C, and iron, and a good way to get potassium and calcium.

Super Start
MENU—DAY 7

BREAKFAST
1 Ounce Cereal Choice
1 Small Bunch Grapes
1 Cup Skim Milk
Coffee, Tea, or Free Drink

ANYTIME SNACK
2 Slices Rye Bread
Coffee, Tea, or Free Drink

LUNCH
*1 Container Yogurt **plus** Pectin*
*Free Salad **plus** Zero Dressing*
2 Pieces Wasa Crispbread
Free Drink

DINNER
*1 Cup Tomato Juice **plus** Pectin*
6 Ounces Broiled Flounder
¾ Cup Cooked Tricolor Pasta
1 Cup Steamed Beets
*Free Salad **plus** Zero Dressing*
Coffee, Tea, or Free Drink

P.M. SNACK
4 Ounces Dry or Semi-dry Wine

Try flavoring cottage cheese with any one of the following:

- *1 green onion, white and green parts, chopped or*
- *2–3 radishes, chopped*
- *2 tablespoons chopped green pepper*
- *2 tablespoons chopped parsley*
- *1 chopped tomato or*
- *all of the above!*

Mixed bean salad is available jarred and also at many "deli" counters. It's easy to make, too. Save leftover cooked or canned beans in the freezer. When you've accumulated a few kinds, simply thaw them and combine with a no-oil Italian dressing—easy and delicious!

We eat with our eyes as well as our mouths. A colorful, nicely arranged salad plate is a treat to eat and pretty to look at. Raw carrot and zucchini sticks are beautiful; combine them with colorful Free Salad Fixings for a hearty, balanced salad. The wider the array of colors presented, the wider the variety of vitamins and minerals offered in the meal. Eat a colorful plate!

Super Start
MENU—DAY 8

BREAKFAST
1 Ounce Cereal Choice
½ Papaya
1 Cup Skim Milk
Coffee, Tea, or *Free Drink*

ANYTIME SNACK
1 Bagel
Coffee, Tea, or *Free Drink*

LUNCH
1 Container Yogurt **plus** *Pectin*
Free Salad **plus** *Zero Dressing*
2 Rice Cakes
Free Drink

DINNER
1 Cup Tomato Juice **plus** *Pectin*
1 Cup Low-fat Cottage Cheese
¾ Cup Mixed Bean Salad
1 Cup Raw Carrot and Zucchini Sticks
Free Salad **plus** *Zero Dressing*
Coffee, Tea, or *Free Drink*

P.M. SNACK
1 Medium Pear

Mix ½ teaspoon Worcestershire sauce and 1 teaspoon minced onion into ground beef before broiling.

Barley is a delicious grain that is rich in soluble fiber—the kind of fiber that helps fill you up and also may lower your cholesterol and blood glucose (sugar) levels. Barley is good hot or cold.

FOR A HOT DISH
Cook barley in water flavored with 1 bouillon cube and 1 teaspoon lemon juice. Stir in chopped parsley or chopped celery leaves just before serving.

FOR A COLD DISH
Cook barley and chill. Add 1 small chopped tomato and 1 tablespoon chopped chives; dress with an herb vinegar. Or, add 1 tablespoon chopped red onion and ¼ cup chopped fennel and dress with a no-oil salad dressing of your choice.

Super Start
MENU—DAY 9

BREAKFAST
1 Ounce Cereal Choice
1 Cup Cubed Casaba Melon
1 Cup Skim Milk
Coffee, Tea, or Free Drink

ANYTIME SNACK
1 English Muffin
Coffee, Tea, or Free Drink

LUNCH
*1 Container Yogurt **plus** Pectin*
*Free Salad **plus** Zero Dressing*
3 Pieces Norwegian Crispbread
Free Drink

DINNER
*1 Cup Tomato Juice **plus** Pectin*
3 Ounces Broiled Ground Round (Beef) Patty
¾ Cup Cooked Barley
1 Cup Steamed Carrots
*Free Salad **plus** Zero Dressing*
Coffee, Tea, or Free Drink

P.M. SNACK
4 Ounces Dry or Semi-dry Wine

BROILED GRAPEFRUIT

For a change from cold fruit for breakfast: *Spread grapefruit with 1 teaspoon diet apple jelly and broil 2–3 minutes. Or, microwave for 30 seconds on medium.*

TIP ▬▬▬▬▬▬▬▬▬▬▬▬▬▬▬▬▬▬▬▬▬▬▬▬▬▬▬▬▬▬

OVEN-ROASTED POTATOES

For a change from boiled or steamed potatoes: *Scrub a large baking potato and cut it into 8 chunks. Place the chunks on a nonstick baking dish, skin-side down; spray lightly with cooking spray. Sprinkle with a little seasoned pepper and paprika for color and zip. Bake at 350 degrees for 30 minutes or until fork tender and lightly browned.*

TIP ▬▬▬▬▬▬▬▬▬▬▬▬▬▬▬▬▬▬▬▬▬▬▬▬▬▬▬▬▬▬

Deep yellow fruits and vegetables and green leafy vegetables are all low in fat and rich in beta-carotene. Research shows that people who eat these fruits and vegetables often can reduce their risk for some types of cancer. Today's menu includes spinach; add other choices high in beta-carotene to your Free Salad at lunch.

Super Start
MENU—DAY 10

BREAKFAST
1 Ounce Cereal Choice
1 Medium Pink Grapefruit
1 Cup Skim Milk
Coffee, Tea, or Free Drink

ANYTIME SNACK
2 Slices Rye Toast
Coffee, Tea, or Free Drink

LUNCH
*1 Container Yogurt **plus** Pectin*
*Free Salad **plus** Zero Dressing*
2 Pieces Melba Toast
Free Drink

DINNER
*1 Cup Tomato Juice **plus** Pectin*
6 Ounces Broiled Halibut
3/4 Cup Roasted Potatoes
1 Cup Steamed Spinach
*Free Salad **plus** Zero Dressing*
Coffee, Tea, or Free Drink

P.M. SNACK
1/2 Cup Fruit Cocktail

Before broiling ground turkey: *Mix in 1 tablespoon chopped parsley, ¹/₄ teaspoon dried dill, and a pinch of nutmeg.*

TOMATO JUICE COCKTAIL

The following is a list of ideas for adding flavor and texture to your dinner tomato juice cocktail. *During Super Start you add 1 tablespoon powdered pectin to your tomato juice cocktail, along with any "zip" you like. Stir in both with a tall, crisp stalk of celery or cucumber.*

USE A DASH OF

Basil, dried	Garlic powder	Onion juice
Cayenne pepper	Hot pepper sauce	Soy sauce
Celery powder	Lemon Pepper	Tabasco
Chili powder	Marjoram, dried	

USE A TEASPOON OF

Beef stock	Lemon juice	Poultry stock
Dill, fresh	Lime juice	Salsa
Horseradish, grated	Parsley, fresh chopped	Tarragon, fresh

USE A TABLESPOON OF

Cucumber, grated	Pepper, green chopped	Scallion rings
Onion, grated	Pepper, yellow chopped	Sweet onion, chopped

Super Start
MENU—DAY 11

BREAKFAST
1 Ounce Cereal Choice
1 Cup Cubed Honeydew Melon
1 Cup Skim Milk
Coffee, Tea, or Free Drink

ANYTIME SNACK
1 Bagel
Coffee, Tea, or Free Drink

LUNCH
1 Container Yogurt plus Pectin
Free Salad plus Zero Dressing
4 Pieces Cracklebread
Free Drink

DINNER
1 Cup Tomato Juice plus Pectin
3 Ounces Broiled Lean Ground Turkey Patty
1 Cup Boiled Parslied New Potato
1 Cup Steamed Lima Beans
Free Salad plus Zero Dressing
Coffee, Tea, or Free Drink

P.M. SNACK
15 Fresh Cherries

As a group, melons are one of the most nutritious fruits. All varieties have substantial levels of potassium and vitamin C, with little or no fat. Cantaloupes contain good amounts of folic acid (a B-vitamin) and vitamin A.

Most people do not know how to select a ripe, tasty melon. The following tips will help.

Cantaloupe is ready to eat when the netting on the surface is thick and coarse and stands out like relief work; it should have a pleasant odor and yield to a slight pressure at the blossom end (opposite the stem end).

Casaba is ready to eat when the hard rind is a golden-yellow color and there is a softening at the blossom end; there is no aroma to this melon.

Crenshaw is ready to eat when the rind is a deep golden-yellow color and the entire surface yields to slight pressure; it has a pleasant aroma.

Honeydew is ready to eat when it has a faint aroma, slight softening at the blossom end and there are loose seeds when shaken.

Persian is ready to eat when it has a fine brown netting imposed on a green background and a pleasant aroma; it will yield slightly to pressure at the blossom end.

Super Start
MENU—DAY 12

BREAKFAST
1 Ounce Cereal Choice
1½ Cups Strawberries
1 Cup Skim Milk
Coffee, Tea, or Free Drink

ANYTIME SNACK
2 Slices Pumpernickel Bread
Coffee, Tea, or Free Drink

LUNCH
*1 Container Yogurt **plus** Pectin*
*Free Salad **plus** Zero Dressing*
2 Rice Cakes
Free Drink

DINNER
*1 Cup Tomato Juice **plus** Pectin*
6 Ounces Broiled Cod
¾ Cup Cooked Spinach Pasta
1 Cup Steamed Carrots
*Free Salad **plus** Zero Dressing*
Coffee, Tea, or Free Drink

P.M. SNACK
¼ Persian Melon

CHICKEN BREAST WITH PASTA

Poach a boneless chicken breast in 1 cup simmering water to which you have added 1 teaspoon powdered chicken bouillon, 1 tablespoon chopped onion, and ¼ teaspoon dried dillweed (or 1 tablespoon chopped fresh dillweed). After 10 minutes, when chicken is nearly done, add ¼ cup uncooked pasta. Continue cooking till pasta is firm, about 10 minutes.

There are two main varieties of peaches: clingstone (the peach flesh *clings* to the pit) and freestone (the pit is easily separated from the flesh, which is softer). Nectarines, "peaches without fuzz," are in fact a variety of peach with smooth skin and firmer flesh.

If fresh peaches aren't available, canned peaches are a real convenience. Most canned fruit can be found in water-packed, juice-packed, and syrup-packed varieties. Juice- or water-packed are better choices because they are more tender and taste more like real fruit.

Super Start
MENU—DAY 13

BREAKFAST
1 Ounce Cereal Choice
1 Peach
1 Cup Skim Milk
Coffee, Tea, or Free Drink

ANYTIME SNACK
1 Bagel
Coffee, Tea, or Free Drink

LUNCH
*1 Container Yogurt **plus** Pectin*
*Free Salad **plus** Zero Dressing*
2 Rice Cakes
Free Drink

DINNER
*1 Cup Tomato Juice **plus** Pectin*
4 Ounces Poached Boneless Chicken Breast
3/4 Cup Cooked Orzo (Rice-shaped Pasta)
1 Cup Steamed Mixed Wax and Green Beans
*Free Salad **plus** Zero Dressing*
Coffee, Tea, or Free Drink

P.M. SNACK
2 Small Figs

TASTY BAKED PORK

Combine 1 teaspoon soy sauce, 1 teaspoon diet grape jelly, 1 tablespoon sherry or cider vinegar, and ½ teaspoon ground ginger. Brush on one pork tenderloin before baking.

Pork has a reputation for being fatty and hard to digest. Neither is true.

Pork tenderloin is an excellent low-fat choice; 3 ounces has only 4 grams of fat. Canadian bacon and fresh ham are other lean pork choices. Choices high in fat are bacon (1 strip has 3 grams of fat) and spareribs (a 3-ounce serving has a whopping 26 grams of fat).

Super Start
MENU—DAY 14

BREAKFAST
1 Ounce Cereal Choice
4 Small Apricots
1 Cup Skim Milk
Coffee, Tea, or Free Drink

ANYTIME SNACK
2 Slices French Bread
Coffee, Tea, or Free Drink

LUNCH
*1 Container Yogurt **plus** Pectin*
*Free Salad **plus** Zero Dressing*
2 Rice Cakes
Free Drink

DINNER
*1 Cup Tomato Juice **plus** Pectin*
4 Ounces Baked Pork Tenderloin
1 Medium Baked Sweet Potato
1 Cup Steamed Corn
*Free Salad **plus** Zero Dressing*
Coffee, Tea, or Free Drink

P.M. SNACK
*4 Ounces Dry **or** Semi-dry Wine*

STEAMED SHRIMP

To dress up steamed shrimp, serve with curry sauce: *Simply mix 1 table-spoon diet apricot jelly, ¼ teaspoon curry powder, and 1 teaspoon lemon juice. Brush on steamed shrimp.*

Shrimp is very low in fat: 3 ounces has only 1 gram.

You've probably heard, however, that shrimp is high in cholesterol. This is not entirely true. Older methods used to measure the amount of cholesterol in shrimp and other shellfish were not accurate. More recent estimates show that there's less cholesterol in shrimp and some other shellfish than was once believed. Shrimp is a good occasional choice, but keep in mind that although a 3-ounce portion of shrimp is very low in fat, it still has double the cholesterol found in 3 ounces of beef.

Super Start
MENU—DAY 15

BREAKFAST
1 Ounce Cereal Choice
1 Large Orange
1 Cup Skim Milk
Coffee, Tea, or Free Drink

ANYTIME SNACK
1 Hard Roll
Coffee, Tea, or Free Drink

LUNCH
1 Container Yogurt **plus** *Pectin*
Free Salad **plus** *Zero Dressing*
2 Pieces Melba Toast
Free Drink

DINNER
1 Cup Tomato Juice **plus** *Pectin*
5 Ounces Steamed Shrimp
3/4 Cup Steamed Rice
1 Cup Steamed Green Peas
Free Salad **plus** *Zero Dressing*
Coffee, Tea, or Free Drink

P.M. SNACK
2 Cups Air-popped Popcorn

FOR A HOT MEAL
Combine ³⁄₄ cup hot cooked pasta with 1 tablespoon picante sauce or mild salsa, 1 teaspoon lemon juice, and 1 cup steamed artichokes.

FOR A COLD MEAL
Combine tuna (canned or fresh broiled), pasta, and artichoke hearts with Free Salad ingredients and Zero Dressing for a large, satisfying salad dinner.

Choose tuna in water for much less fat.

3 ounces tuna canned in oil has 7 grams of fat
3 ounces tuna canned in water has 2 grams of fat

Super Start
MENU—DAY 16

BREAKFAST
1 Ounce Cereal Choice
2 Clementines
1 Cup Skim Milk
Coffee, Tea, or Free Drink

ANYTIME SNACK
1 Bagel
Coffee, Tea, or Free Drink

LUNCH
1 Container Yogurt **plus** Pectin
Free Salad **plus** Zero Dressing
3 Pieces Norwegian Crispbread
Free Drink

DINNER
1 Cup Tomato Juice **plus** Pectin
$1/2$ Cup Tuna
$3/4$ Cup Boiled Tricolor Pasta
1 Cup Steamed Artichoke Hearts
Free Salad **plus** Zero Dressing
Coffee, Tea, or Free Drink

P.M. SNACK
1 Medium Apple

TIP ▬▬

Before serving beans: *Add 1 tablespoon salsa and 2 tablespoons chopped raw celery. This adds lots of crunch and flavor, but no fat.*

TIP ▬▬

Thinly sliced roast beef is available in packages or at the "deli" counter in most supermarkets.

It can be served hot or cold for dinner. To warm the sliced roast beef, put it in a steamer basket and heat, covered, for a minute or two over simmering water.

Although beef is higher in cholesterol than chicken or fish, it is still a lean Main Dish choice, with only 6 grams of fat in 3 ounces. Eating lean cuts of beef in moderate serving sizes (3 to 4 ounces) is fine. Beef supplies protein and minerals like zinc and iron.

Super Start
MENU—DAY 17

BREAKFAST
1 Ounce Cereal Choice
⅙ Crenshaw Melon
1 Cup Skim Milk
Coffee, Tea, or Free Drink

ANYTIME SNACK
1 English Muffin
Coffee, Tea, or Free Drink

LUNCH
1 Container Yogurt **plus** *Pectin*
Free Salad **plus** *Zero Dressing*
4 Pieces Cracklebread
Free Drink

DINNER
1 Cup Tomato Juice **plus** *Pectin*
3 Ounces Thinly Sliced Lean Roast Beef
½ Cup Cooked Cannellini Beans
1 Cup Cooked Sugar Snap Peas
Free Salad **plus** *Zero Dressing*
Coffee, Tea, or Free Drink

P.M. SNACK
4 Ounces Dry or Semi-dry Wine

FOR A LOW-FAT MAIN DISH WITH AN ITALIAN FLAVOR

Brown ground round in a nonstick skillet until it has lost all its pink color; drain off any fat that has accumulated in the pan. Add stewed tomatoes, which are tasty and low in fat, along with 1 teaspoon chopped fresh basil and a pinch of garlic. Cover and simmer 5 minutes or until thoroughly heated. Serve over cooked spaghetti.

If you enjoy pasta, you'll love the delicious whole-wheat varieties imported from Italy that are becoming increasingly available at health-food stores or in supermarkets.

Whole-wheat pasta cooks to a creamy light-brown color and is richer in vitamins, minerals, and fiber than regular varieties.

Newer varieties—containing oat bran, amaranth, triticale, and other less familiar whole grains—are also available. Experiment with these wholesome, nutritious pastas to see which you like best.

Super Start
MENU—DAY 18

BREAKFAST
1 Ounce Cereal Choice
4 Prunes
1 Cup Skim Milk
Coffee, Tea, or Free Drink

ANYTIME SNACK
2 Slices Rye Bread
Coffee, Tea, or Free Drink

LUNCH
1 Container Yogurt **plus** *Pectin*
Free Salad **plus** *Zero Dressing*
2 Rice Cakes
Free Drink

DINNER
1 Cup Tomato Juice **plus** *Pectin*
3 Ounces Broiled Ground Round (Beef) Patty
3/4 Cup Cooked Spaghetti
1 Cup Stewed Tomatoes
Free Salad **plus** *Zero Dressing*
Coffee, Tea, or Free Drink

P.M. SNACK
1 Large Persimmon

POACHED SOLE

For a delicious change from broiled: *Place sole in a skillet with 1 inch gently simmering water that has been flavored with 2–3 lemon slices, 1/4 cup chopped celery leaves, and a few peppercorns. Simmer gently about 10 minutes, or until fish flakes easily. Remove fish from poaching liquid with a slotted spoon and garnish with paprika and chopped fresh parsley.*

TIP ▬▬▬▬▬▬▬▬▬▬▬▬▬▬▬▬▬▬▬▬▬▬▬▬▬▬▬▬▬▬▬▬▬▬▬▬▬

Fish, especially those from cold water, are sources of Omega-3 fatty acids, popularly referred to as "fish oil." Research has shown that the polyunsaturated fatty acids found in fish may have many health benefits: They are being used to treat migraine headaches, arthritis, and high blood lipids (fats). You can buy fish oils in capsule form, but experts recommend that it's safer to get your Omega-3s directly from fish. You can do this easily by eating fish two or three times a week.

Super Start
MENU—DAY 19

BREAKFAST
1 Ounce Cereal Choice
1 Cup Raspberries
1 Cup Skim Milk
Coffee, Tea, or Free Drink

ANYTIME SNACK
1 Bagel
Coffee, Tea, or Free Drink

LUNCH
*1 Container Yogurt **plus** Pectin*
*Free Salad **plus** Zero Dressing*
4 Pieces Cracklebread
Free Drink

DINNER
*1 Cup Tomato Juice **plus** Pectin*
6 Ounces Broiled Sole
1 large Baked Potato
1 Cup Steamed Italian Green Beans
*Free Salad **plus** Zero Dressing*
Coffee, Tea, or Free Drink

P.M. SNACK
2 Medium Plums

Try mixing cooked wild rice and cooked white rice together for added color and flavor.

FOR TASTY BAKED SQUASH
Fill cavity with 1 teaspoon of any flavor diet jelly; sprinkle with cinnamon. Place in baking dish and pour in ¹/₂ inch water to surround squash. Bake at 350 degrees for 45 minutes or until squash is tender when flesh is pierced with a fork. To save time, squash can be microwaved in less than 10 minutes.

Butternut, acorn, summer, pattypan, spaghetti, zucchini, and turban are some of the many kinds of squashes available at different times during the year.

All varieties contain only a trace of fat and are good sources of fiber. Winter squash—butternut, acorn, Hubbard, and pumpkin—are more nutritious than summer squash. They have twice as much potassium and ten times more vitamin A.

Squash flowers can also be eaten, but they're usually battered and deep fried, so they wind up high in fat. A far better use for these edible blossoms is to use them to decorate a salad or as a garnish on a dinner plate.

Super Start
MENU—DAY 20

BREAKFAST

1 Ounce Cereal Choice

2 Tangerines

1 Cup Skim Milk

Coffee, Tea, or Free Drink

ANYTIME SNACK

1 Bagel

Coffee, Tea, or Free Drink

LUNCH

1 Container Yogurt plus Pectin

Free Salad plus Zero Dressing

2 Rice Cakes

Free Drink

DINNER

1 Cup Tomato Juice plus Pectin

4 Ounces Roast Turkey (without skin)

3/4 Cup Boiled White and Wild Rice

1/2 Medium Baked Acorn Squash

Free Salad plus Zero Dressing

Coffee, Tea, or Free Drink

P.M. SNACK

4 Ounces Dry or Semi-dry Wine

TIP ▰▰

Select lentils often; high in soluble fiber, they will help lower your cholesterol. To add a little flavor to this humble but wholesome bean: *Combine 1 tablespoon tomato paste, 1 teaspoon lemon juice, and 1 tablespoon chopped raw onion with cooked lentils.*

TIP ▰▰

For a great no-fat flavor boost, try preparing an Italian "gremolata," a mixture of seasonings which can be used to flavor meat, fish, poultry, or salads. Here's one of many variations for this classic seasoning mixture.

GREMOLATA

Makes 12 Teaspoons

2 tablespoons grated lemon rind
2 teaspoons finely chopped fresh rosemary or 1 teaspoon dried rosemary
1 tablespoon finely chopped parsley
2 cloves garlic, chopped fine

Thoroughly combine all ingredients. To store gremolata, refrigerate in a tightly covered dish or place in a resealable plastic bag and freeze. This mixture will keep in the refrigerator for several days but can be kept frozen for up to a month.

Sprinkle on meat, fish, or poultry just before cooking is complete or just before serving; let stand a few minutes to absorb flavor.

Super Start
MENU—DAY 21

BREAKFAST
1 Ounce Cereal Choice
2 Tablespoons Raisins
1 Cup Skim Milk
Coffee, Tea, or Free Drink

ANYTIME SNACK
2 Slices Whole Wheat Toast
Coffee, Tea, or Free Drink

LUNCH
1 Container Yogurt *plus* Pectin
Free Salad *plus* Zero Dressing
2 Rice Cakes
Free Drink

DINNER
1 Cup Tomato Juice *plus* Pectin
3 Ounces Broiled Beef Sirloin
1/2 Cup Cooked Lentils
1 Cup Steamed Asparagus Tips
Free Salad *plus* Zero Dressing
Coffee, Tea, or Free Drink

P.M. SNACK
1/4 Medium Cantaloupe

TIP ▬▬▬▬▬▬▬▬▬▬▬▬▬▬▬▬▬▬▬▬▬▬▬▬▬▬▬▬▬▬▬▬▬▬▬▬▬▬▬

Brown rice takes longer to cook than white rice. To cut the cooking time in half, mix the rice and water together to soak for about an hour before you plan to cook the rice. You can even do this in the morning before you leave for work. Soaking rice in the water in which it will be cooked does not reduce its nutritional value, since all the water will be absorbed into the rice during cooking.

TIP ▬▬▬▬▬▬▬▬▬▬▬▬▬▬▬▬▬▬▬▬▬▬▬▬▬▬▬▬▬▬▬▬▬▬▬▬▬▬▬

BEFORE COOKING RICE
Add 1 teaspoon powdered vegetable broth (¹/₂ small vegetable broth cube), 1 tablespoon chopped chives, 2 tablespoons chopped celery, and 2 teaspoons chopped fresh basil. Cook rice according to package directions.

TIP ▬▬▬▬▬▬▬▬▬▬▬▬▬▬▬▬▬▬▬▬▬▬▬▬▬▬▬▬▬▬▬▬▬▬▬▬▬▬▬

Brown rice is about 10 percent rice bran. Recent research has shown that rice bran, like oat bran, helps lower blood cholesterol when eaten regularly.

Super Start
MENU—Day 22

BREAKFAST
1 Ounce Cereal Choice
1 Cup Blueberries
1 Cup Skim Milk
Coffee, Tea, or Free Drink

ANYTIME SNACK
2 Slices Pumpernickel Bread
Coffee, Tea, or Free Drink

LUNCH
1 Container Yogurt **plus** *Pectin*
Free Salad **plus** *Zero Dressing*
2 Pieces Wasa Crispbread
Free Drink

DINNER
1 Cup Tomato Juice **plus** *Pectin*
4 Ounces Baked Perch
¾ Cup Steamed Brown Rice
1 Cup Steamed Green Beans
Free Salad **plus** *Zero Dressing*
Coffee, Tea, or Free Drink

P.M. SNACK
2 Cups Air-popped Popcorn

For added flavor, after skinless chicken is almost cooked, brush with one of the following and continue cooking till done:

- *1 tablespoon mustard mixed with 1 teaspoon lemon juice*
- *1 tablespoon mustard mixed with 1 teaspoon diet apricot jelly*
- *1 tablespoon salsa*

To add more flavor to nutty-tasting brown rice.

FOR A HOT DISH
Mushrooms are a wonderful addition: *Add 2 sliced mushrooms to the rice during the last 10 minutes of cooking. Another easy way to prepare mushrooms without any added fat is in the microwave. Wash and slice the mushrooms and place in a covered, vented dish. Cook on medium heat for 2 minutes. Stir the cooked mushrooms into the cooked brown rice. You can also use this trick to add mushrooms to any dish.*

FOR A COLD DISH
For a change, try a Red Rice Salad: *Cook and cool rice. Add 2 tablespoons raspberry vinegar, 1 tablespoon chopped pimiento, and 1 tablespoon chopped red pepper. Serve on a bed of radicchio and garnish with red-onion rings.*

Super Start
MENU—DAY 23

BREAKFAST
1 Ounce Cereal Choice
1 Small Banana
1 Cup Skim Milk
Coffee, Tea, or Free Drink

ANYTIME SNACK
1 Bagel
Coffee, Tea, or Free Drink

LUNCH
*1 Container Yogurt **plus** Pectin*
*Free Salad **plus** Zero Dressing*
2 Rice Cakes
Free Drink

DINNER
*1 Cup Tomato Juice **plus** Pectin*
1 Skinned and Roasted Chicken Leg and Thigh
3/4 Cup Cooked Brown Rice
1 Cup Steamed Cauliflower
*Free Salad **plus** Zero Dressing*
Coffee, Tea, or Free Drink

P.M. SNACK
1 Cup Watermelon

TIP ━━

Instead of cooking zucchini plain, try this idea: *Cut a medium-size zucchini in half lengthwise, spray each half lightly with olive oil cooking spray, and sprinkle with dried oregano and pepper. Bake at 350 degrees for 20 minutes or until lightly browned and tender.*

TIP ━━

Most of you have eaten familiar grains like rice, wheat, and oats, but there are still many more to try. All grains are very low in fat; most contain only a trace in a usual serving. Be adventurous! Try some of the following interesting, flavorful, and nutritious varieties.

Amaranth, called the "grain of the gods" by the Aztecs, is a good source of protein and calcium; also look for cereals with this grain.

Wheat berries are the original form of the wheat grain that is ground into flour; wheat berries require long cooking time, but the result is a chewy, nutty grain that can be served like rice.

Cracked Wheat (bulgur) is produced by cracking toasted wheat berries; it softens by soaking in a matter of minutes, so it's perfect as the base of a cold grain salad.

Kasha (buckwheat groats) is higher in protein than most grains; this one grows around the world and has a pleasant hearty flavor.

Super Start
MENU—DAY 24

BREAKFAST
1 Ounce Cereal Choice
1 Tangelo
1 Cup Skim Milk
Coffee, Tea, or Free Drink

ANYTIME SNACK
2 Slices French Bread
Coffee, Tea, or Free Drink

LUNCH
1 Container Yogurt plus Pectin
Free Salad plus Zero Dressing
4 Pieces Cracklebread
Free Drink

DINNER
1 Cup Tomato Juice plus Pectin
6 Ounces Baked Scallops
3/4 Cup Steamed Buckwheat Groats (Kasha)
1/2 Medium Baked Zucchini
Free Salad plus Zero Dressing
Coffee, Tea, or Free Drink

P.M. SNACK
4 Ounces Dry or Semi-dry Wine

For added flavor, brush ground veal patty, before broiling, with a mixture of 1 teaspoon mustard, a few drops of Worcestershire sauce, and a pinch of ground ginger.

Without using a scale, you can use these simple guidelines to estimate a serving of meat, fish, or poultry.

Boneless: A 4-ounce portion is approximately the size of the palm of your hand and as thick as your hand where the palm meets the smallest finger. A 3-ounce portion is the size and thickness of a deck of cards.

Chopped: A ½-cup measure is a good approximation for a 3- to 4-ounce portion of chopped meat, cubed meat, or flaked cooked fish.

Bone-in: A closed fist approximates the size of half a chicken breast, which has about 3 ounces of meat on it.

Super Start
MENU—Day 25

BREAKFAST
1 Ounce Cereal Choice
1 Cup Blackberries
1 Cup Skim Milk
Coffee, Tea, or Free Drink

ANYTIME SNACK
2 Slices Rye Toast
Coffee, Tea, or Free Drink

LUNCH
*1 Container Yogurt **plus** Pectin*
*Free Salad **plus** Zero Dressing*
2 Rice Cakes
Free Drink

DINNER
*1 Cup Tomato Juice **plus** Pectin*
4 Ounces Broiled Ground Veal Patty
¾ Cup Cooked Sweet Potato
1 Cup Steamed Mixed Vegetables
*Free Salad **plus** Zero Dressing*
Coffee, Tea, or Free Drink

P.M. SNACK
8 Dried Apricot Halves

SLICED LAMB WITH TABOULEH

To make a simple low-fat tabouleh salad: *Soak ½ cup bulgur in ¾ cup boiling water for about 20 minutes. Squeeze out water and then flavor bulgur with ½ tteaspoon salt, 1 tablespoon lemon juice, 1 tablespoon fresh chopped mint, 2 tablespoons chopped parsley, and ¼ cup chopped cucumber. Serve with sliced lamb.*

TIP ▬▬▬▬▬▬▬▬▬▬▬▬▬▬▬▬▬▬▬▬▬▬▬▬▬▬▬▬▬▬▬▬▬▬▬

If you enjoy lamb, the best cut is lean boneless leg with 6 grams of fat in a 3-ounce portion. A boneless shoulder cut has 50 percent more fat, or 9 grams in a 3-ounce portion. Ground lamb patties have 16 grams of fat in 3 ounces.

TIP ▬▬▬▬▬▬▬▬▬▬▬▬▬▬▬▬▬▬▬▬▬▬▬▬▬▬▬▬▬▬▬▬▬▬▬

Select whole-grain breads whenever you can. They have only a trace of fat and more vitamins, minerals, and fiber than white bread.

Super Start
MENU—DAY 26

BREAKFAST
1 Ounce Cereal Choice
1 Large Nectarine
1 Cup Skim Milk
Coffee, Tea, or Free Drink

ANYTIME SNACK
1 Bagel
Coffee, Tea, or Free Drink

LUNCH
1 Container Yogurt plus Pectin
Free Salad plus Zero Dressing
2 Pieces Wasa Crispbread
Free Drink

DINNER
1 Cup Tomato Juice plus Pectin
3 Ounces Boneless Roast Leg of Lamb
¾ Cup Cooked Bulgur
1 Cup Steamed Brussels Sprouts
Free Salad plus Zero Dressing
Coffee, Tea, or Free Drink

P.M. SNACK
4 Ounces Dry or Semi-dry Wine

For a change, why not bake an apple and have a warm after-dinner snack with a fragrant cup of hot tea?

BAKED APPLE

Core an apple and place it in a small glass dish. Fill the apple cavity with 2 teaspoons of diet orange marmalade and a sprinkle of cinnamon. Bake at 350 degrees for 30 to 40 minutes, or until the apple is tender. To microwave, cook for 2 to 3 minutes on medium.

"3-ONION" TURKEY CUTLETS

Poach cutlets for 20 minutes in simmering water to which you have added 4 slices red onion, 4 slices white onion, 2 tablespoons sliced green onion (white and green part), and ¼ teaspoon dried dill. Serve poached onions on top of turkey.

Super Start
MENU—DAY 27

BREAKFAST
1 Ounce Cereal Choice
½ Cup Pineapple
1 Cup Skim Milk
Coffee, Tea, or Free Drink

ANYTIME SNACK
1 English Muffin
Coffee, Tea, or Free Drink

LUNCH
*1 Container Yogurt **plus** Pectin*
*Free Salad **plus** Zero Dressing*
3 Pieces Norwegian Crispbread
Free Drink

DINNER
*1 Cup Tomato Juice **plus** Pectin*
4 Ounces Poached Turkey Breast Cutlet
1 Medium Baked Sweet Potato
1 Cup Chopped Broccoli
*Free Salad **plus** Zero Dressing*
Coffee, Tea, or Free Drink

P.M. SNACK
1 Medium Apple

TASTY FISH

In a rangetop/ovenproof dish, mix ¾ cup water with 1 teaspoon lemon juice. Bring to a boil; add ¼ cup raw rice. Reduce to a simmer and cook 15 minutes. Remove from heat and mix 1 tablespoon chopped onion and 1 tablespoon chopped fresh parsley into rice. Arrange raw red snapper on rice; spray on cooking spray and sprinkle with paprika. Bake at 350 degrees for 15 minutes in a preheated oven.

TIP ▬▬▬▬▬▬▬▬▬▬▬▬▬▬▬▬▬▬▬▬▬▬▬▬▬▬▬▬▬▬▬▬▬▬▬▬

Popcorn is a great snack anytime, but it's especially satisfying when you're trying to lose weight. It offers a lot of chewing and a cup of air-popped corn has only a trace of fat.

Microwave and cheese-flavored popcorns are much higher in fat, with 3 grams or more in a cup. Popcorn that comes in its own pan, ready to pop, usually has added fat or oil, as does prepopped packaged popcorn. Making your own is the best way to control the fat (and the salt).

Super Start
MENU—DAY 28

BREAKFAST
1 Ounce Cereal Choice
½ Cup Mandarin Oranges
1 Cup Skim Milk
Coffee, Tea, or Free Drink

ANYTIME SNACK
1 Bagel
Coffee, Tea, or Free Drink

LUNCH
*1 Container Yogurt **plus** Pectin*
*Free Salad **plus** Zero Dressing*
2 Rice Cakes
Free Drink

DINNER
6 Ounces Baked Red Snapper
¾ Cup Cooked Rice
1 Cup Steamed Yellow Squash
*Free Salad **plus** Zero Dressing*
Coffee, Tea, or Free Drink

P.M. SNACK
2 Cups Air-popped Popcorn

Super Start
FOOD LISTS

These lists make it easier for you to attack your fat. Refer to them whenever your Super Start menu indicates that you have a food choice to make.

During Super Start, use:

Cereal Choices

Yogurt Choices

Lunch Cracker Choices

Dinner Juice Substitutes

Free Salad Fixings

Free Drinks

Super Start Free Sweets

Free Condiments

Super Start CEREAL CHOICES

For Super Start, choose a 1-ounce serving of any one of the following cereals.

100% Bran with Oat Bran   NABISCO
100% Oat Bran   SKINNERS
7-Grain Crunchy   LOMA LINDA
7-Grain No Sugar Added   LOMA LINDA
Cheerios   GENERAL MILLS
Cheerios, Apple Cinnamon   GENERAL MILLS
Cheerios, Honey Nut   GENERAL MILLS
Common Sense Oat Bran   KELLOGG'S
Cracklin' Oat Bran   KELLOGG'S
Fortified Oat Flakes   POST
Honey Bunches of Oats   POST
Hot Bran Hot Cereal   HEALTH VALLEY
Instant Oatmeal   QUAKER
Instant Oatmeal Regular   EREWHON
Instant Oatmeal Regular   RALSTON
Instant Oatmeal with Apples & Cinnamon   QUAKER
Instant Oatmeal with Cinnamon & Spice   RALSTON
Instant Oatmeal with Cinnamon & Spices   QUAKER
Instant Oatmeal with Maple & Brown Sugar   QUAKER
Instant Oatmeal with Maple & Brown Sugar   RALSTON
Irish Oatmeal, Quick Cooking   McCANN'S
Kashi, 5 Bran Instant Cereal   KASHI
Kashi, Lightly Puffed   KASHI
Kashi, the Breakfast Pilaf   KASHI
Nutrific Oatmeal Flakes   KELLOGG'S
Oat Bran   MOTHERS
Oat Bran   QUAKER
Oat Bran Crunch   KOLLIN
Oat Bran Flakes   HEALTH VALLEY
Oat Bran Options   RALSTON
Oat Bran O's   HEALTH VALLEY
Oat Bran O's Fruit & Nuts   HEALTH VALLEY
Oat Bran with Toasted Wheat Germ   EREWHON
Oat Meal   McCANN'S
Oat Squares   QUAKER

Oatmeal Maple Flavor   MAYPO
Oatmeal Raisin Crisp   GENERAL MILLS
Oatmeal Swirlers   GENERAL MILLS
Old Fashioned Oatmeal   QUAKER
Puffed Kashi   KASHI
Quaker Extra Apples & Spice   QUAKER
Quaker Extra Raisins & Cinnamon   QUAKER
Quaker Extra Regular   QUAKER
Quick Oatmeal   RALSTON
Quick Oats   ROMAN MEAL
Regular Oatmeal   RALSTON
Total Instant Oatmeal Regular   GENERAL MILLS
Total Oatmeal Quick   GENERAL MILLS
Wholesome 'n Hearty Instant Oat Bran Hot Cereal   NABISCO
Wholesome 'n Hearty Instant Oat Bran Hot Cereal, Honey   NABISCO
Wholesome 'n Hearty Instant Oat Bran Hot Cereal, Apple Cinnamon
   NABISCO
Wholesome 'n Hearty Oat Bran Hot Cereal   NABISCO

Super Start YOGURT CHOICES

Each of the yogurts listed below is a low-fat choice, containing 2 grams of fat or less per container or 1-cup serving.

AXELROD

Plain	Vanilla

BREYERS LOW-FAT

Blueberry	Pineapple	Strawberry Banana
Peach	Raspberry	

CONTINENTAL NONFAT

Honey Nut Crunch	Plain	Wildberry
Peach	Raspberry	

COLOMBO NONFAT LITE

Banana Strawberry	Peach	Strawberry
Blueberry	Plain	Vanilla
Fruit Cocktail		

Super Start YOGURT CHOICES (*cont.*)

DANNON NON-FAT

Plain

KNUDSON

Lemon	Peach	Strawberry Banana

LA YOGURT 25 NON-FAT

Blueberry	Raspberry	Strawberry Banana
Cherry	Strawberry	

LIGHT N' LIVELY

Black Cherry	Pineapple	Strawberry Banana
Blueberry	Red Raspberry	Strawberry Fruit Cup
Peach	Strawberry	

LITE LINE

Cherry Vanilla	Plain Lowfat Swiss Style	Strawberry
Peach		

NEW COUNTRY

Apple Crisp	Hawaiian Salad	Raspberry Supreme
Blueberry Supreme	Lemon Supreme	Strawberry Banana
Cherry Supreme	Mixed Berries	Strawberry Fruit Cup
French Vanilla	Orange Supreme	Strawberry Supreme
Fruit Crunch	Peaches 'n Cream	

SWEET 'n LOW RIPPLE

Cherry	Raspberry	Strawberry
Peach		

TUSCAN FARMS LOWFAT YOGURT DRINK

All Flavors

WEIGHT WATCHERS

Black Cherry   Blueberry   Raspberry

WEIGHT WATCHERS ULTIMATE

Blueberry   Plain   Strawberry Banana

YOPLAIT 90

Strawberry Banana

YOPLAIT 150

Blueberry   Peach   Strawberry
Cherry   Raspberry   Strawberry Banana

YOPLAIT ORIGINAL

Apple   Cherry   Lemon

Super Start LUNCH CRACKER CHOICES

Cracklebread	4 pieces	Rice cakes, any variety	2 pieces
Melba toast, any variety	2 pieces	Ry Krisp, Seasoned	3 pieces
Norwegian crispbread	3 pieces	Wasa crispbread, any variety	2 pieces
Oat Bran Krisp	2 pieces	Weight Watchers Crispbread	4 pieces
Popcorn, unbuttered	2 cups		

Super Start DINNER JUICE SUBSTITUTES

Beefamato juice   Gazpacho (see   Tomato juice
Celery juice   recipe page 86)   V-8 Juice
Clamato juice   Grapefruit juice

Super Start FREE SALAD FIXINGS

Alfalfa sprouts   Basil, fresh   Bibb lettuce
Arugula   Bean sprouts   Bok choy

Super Start FREE SALAD FIXINGS (*cont.*)

Boston lettuce
Butterhead lettuce
Cabbage
Cabbage, Chinese
Cabbage, red
Cabbage, savoy
Celery
Chard
Chicory
Chives
Cilantro
Cress
Cucumber
Dill, fresh
Endive
Escarole
Fennel

Garden cress
Garlic
Green onions
   (scallions)
Hot peppers
Iceberg lettuce
Kale
Kohlrabi
Looseleaf lettuce
Mint, fresh
Mung bean
   sprouts
Mushrooms
Mustard greens
Onions, red
Onions, Spanish
Onions, Vidalia

Onions, white
Parsley, fresh
Peppers, green
Peppers, red
Peppers, yellow
Pimiento
Radicchio
Radishes
Red-leaf lettuce
Rocket
Romaine lettuce
Sorrel
Shallot
Spinach
Tomato
Watercress

Super Start FREE DRINKS

Club soda
Diet soda
Drink mixes,
   sugar free
Herbal tea

Instant onion
   soup, dry mix
Mineral water
Pero (coffee
   substitute)

Postum (coffee
   substitute)
Seltzer
Seltzer, flavored
Water

Super Start FREE SWEETS

Diet jam
Diet jelly
Sugar-free gelatin

Sugar-free gum
Sugar-free hard
   candy

Sugar substitutes

Super Start FREE CONDIMENTS

Use the following condiments to flavor, garnish, or prepare foods.

Beef broth, cubes or powdered
Butter-flavored sprinkles

Chicken broth, cubes or
   powdered

Chives
Garlic
Ginger root
Gremolata (see page 118)
Herbs, dried (see pages 67–69)
Herbs, fresh (see pages 67–69)
Horseradish
Hot sauce
Ketchup
Lemon
Lemon juice
Lime
Lime juice
Mustard, coarse grain
Mustard, Dijon
Mustard, lemon
Mustard, regular
Mustard, tarragon
No-oil salad dressing
Pepper
Picante sauce
Pickles, dill

Salsa
Salt-free seasoning mixtures
Seasoned pepper
Shallot
Soy sauce, regular
Soy sauce, light
Spices (see pages 67–69)
Tabasco sauce
Tamari
Tomato paste
Teriyaki sauce
Vegetable broth, cubes or powdered
Vinegar
Vinegar, balsamic
Vinegar, cider
Vinegar, herb flavored
Vinegar, raspberry
Vinegar, rice
Vinegar, tarragon
Vinegar, wine
Watermelon rind pickles
Worcestershire sauce
Zero Dressing (see page 78)

8 *Getting Ahead*
FAT ATTACK PLAN PHASE TWO

You should be *very* proud of yourself. You're Getting Ahead already! If this is where you're starting your Fat Attack, you don't have too much weight to lose. And by the time you've achieved your target weight— twenty-eight days on Getting Ahead should do it—you'll be on the road to better health as well.

If you've just finished Super Start and you're about to start your second twenty-eight days on the Fat Attack Plan, the first thing you should do is take a look in the mirror and tell yourself what a great job you've done. You've lost twelve to fifteen pounds—quite an achievement! Now get ready to shift gears, move into the next phase of the Fat Attack Plan, and lose five to ten more pounds. Getting Ahead will actually provide you with more fat foods than you've had during the last four weeks on Super Start, but your fat intake will still be low enough to ensure weight loss and improved health. If you don't need to review why and you're eager to get going, move right to page 144 now, and start learning how to "track your fat" so that you'll be able to set up your delicious Getting Ahead menus.

If This Is Where You're Beginning

Whatever your weight-loss goal, Getting Ahead will help you achieve it. But for those of you beginning the Fat Attack Plan with Getting Ahead, your primary goal will be lowering your health risks while losing five to ten pounds. Over the next twenty-eight days, your total cholesterol will go down, as will your triglycerides. Your blood glucose (sugar) will also drop as you lose weight, reducing your risk for diabetes.

Why Lower Your Fat Intake?

All of these positive changes will be accomplished by doing just one thing: keeping the amount of fat in your diet low. Each day that you're on Getting Ahead you'll be eating less fat than you have been eating for a long time (unless you've already been on Super Start). You'll quickly see what attacking your fat can do for your looks . . . and for your health! By eating less fat you'll automatically lose weight, lower your cholesterol, and reduce your overall health risks.

Why? First of all, fat is an extremely rich source of calories, so when you eat fatty foods you're giving your body a hefty dose of "energy" to burn. But your body looks to carbohydrate and protein calories to burn before it looks to fat calories; therefore, many of these fat calories are just stored away as body fat. Unfortunately, the fat you eat is also much more easily converted into body fat than the carbohydrates and protein you eat. So the fat you eat will almost always become the fat you wear.

In simpler terms: If you eat more fat, you'll be fatter; if you eat less fat, you'll be thinner. But if you eat less *fat,* you can eat *more* carbohydrates and protein—and still lose weight!

LESS FAT MEANS LOWER CHOLESTEROL

Dietary fat (the fat in foods) also provides your body with the raw material it needs to manufacture cholesterol. You may be one of those people who've already stopped eating eggs and steak, but your cholesterol is still high. What's happening? Your body is manufacturing cholesterol from the *other* fats in your diet. The solution? The simplest way to lower cholesterol and keep it down is to eat less of *all* kinds of fat, not just the ones often found in red meat and dairy products. How? By Getting Ahead on the Fat Attack Plan.

You won't have to count calories. You won't have to do much menu planning either, if you don't want to. All you'll have to do is track the amount of fat in your diet each day.

You'll do this by following a basic Menu Pattern to which *you* add some fat. You'll select from a list of fat-food choices and create menus to your liking that include the fat foods you've chosen. But by keeping the amount of fat you eat within the Getting Ahead guidelines, you'll have the assurance that you'll lower your cholesterol and your other health risks, *and* lose weight, too.

28 Days to Success

You'll do all this in just *twenty-eight* days of very good eating, and with each day on Getting Ahead you'll be closer to achieving your target weight and to lowering your health risks. Many of our clients find that a good way to watch their progress is to record each day they're on Getting Ahead. They do it by marking "Day 1," "Day 2," "Day 3," and so on, right on the calendar on their kitchen wall, or with the help of a list of days, like this one, on which they cross off each Getting Ahead day they complete.

---

28 DAYS TO SUCCESS

Day 1	Day 8	Day 15	Day 22
Day 2	Day 9	Day 16	Day 23
Day 3	Day 10	Day 17	Day 24
Day 4	Day 11	Day 18	Day 25
Day 5	Day 12	Day 19	Day 26
Day 6	Day 13	Day 20	Day 27
Day 7	Day 14	Day 21	Day 28

BUT WHAT IF...?

What if something special comes up during the next twenty-eight days and you can't eat your Getting Ahead menu that day? Don't worry. Simply go ahead and enjoy the special event, *but on that day don't mark your calendar.* The next day, pick up where you left off. *One day* will not sabotage the success you've achieved so far, as long as it's just one day. Thin people do it all the time: They enjoy special foods once in a while, then go back to making sensible food choices the rest of the time.

Often a dieter will use a day when they "cheated" as an excuse to stop dieting. They claim they have no willpower: They can't stick to anything too long, foods they love "call out" to them and they just can't resist. The Fat Attack Plan is set up to help you through all those pitfalls.

For one thing, when you're eating according to the Fat Attack Plan, you can't cheat—because no foods are forbidden! It's okay to stray from the Menu Pattern on occasion. But guess what? Even on Getting Ahead you may not be "straying." If certain foods are just crying out your name, you don't have to turn your back on them, because you'll find that many of the foods you love are options you can add to your Getting Ahead menus. You simply work the right amount of them into your plan for the day. But how do you know how much of these foods you can have?

Tracking Your Fat

In Getting Ahead, you attack your fat by "tracking your fat." Fat in food is measured by weight in grams. Butter, a high-fat food, is almost all fat—one little tablespoon has twelve grams! Broccoli, on the other hand, is a low-fat food—one cup has less than a gram. But if you put the butter *on* the broccoli—what's happened to the low-fat food? Zoom. It's now a high-fat food.

When you're on the Getting Ahead phase of the Fat Attack Plan, you'll be keeping track of the fat you eat each day. You'll be personalizing your daily menus by adding fifteen grams of fat a day to a basic Menu Pattern. You'll select those fifteen grams—of any fat food you'd like—from the list of Getting Ahead Fat Choices on pages 222–23.

The basic Menu Pattern already contains some fat in the form of protein foods, like meat, with lesser amounts from other foods; but you'll get to add even more from the long list of nearly seventy choices. You can decide to use all fifteen grams of fat at one time, or spread your choices out through the course of the day. Not only will you have the fun of personalizing your diet, but you'll learn about making sensible fat-food choices at the same time.

If you love peanut butter, have some—perhaps on toast as a snack. You can see from the Fat Choices list that one tablespoon of peanut butter has eight grams of fat. Since you'll be choosing fifteen grams of fat to add to your basic Menu Pattern each day, you'll still have seven grams of fat left to use that day, after eating your peanut butter. You can use it on anything you want—even more peanut butter!

Here's another example. Even though you know it's better to use low-fat milk most of the time, you'd just love to start the day with a cup of coffee with cream. When you check the Fat Choices list you see that two tablespoons (one ounce) of half-and-half contains four grams of fat. Subtract that from the fifteen grams you get each day and you still have eleven grams of fat left to enjoy any way you'd like.

As you become more familiar with the Fat Choices list, you'll learn which foods are very high in fat and which ones are low. Obviously, you can eat much larger portions of the lower-fat foods; the high-fat ones can be used as treats. But they *can* be used. That's the fun, and the reward, of Getting Ahead.

Getting Ahead with Thin Habits

Back in chapter 4 we talked about getting into some new "Thin Habits." These are the new ways of choosing foods and eating them that will help you lose weight and keep it off.

If you've already been through Super Start, you've already learned several Thin Habits. You'll practice these in Getting Ahead and learn some new ones, too. If you're starting with Getting Ahead, you'll get a good lesson right here. By incorporating these Thin Habits into the way you eat—now and in the future—you'll acquire the tools you'll need to reach and maintain your target weight, to lower your health risks, and to delay the onset of serious illness. And, of course, you'll take these Thin Habits with you when you move on to healthy, low-fat living "In Control."

GETTING AHEAD THIN HABITS

- Choose low-fat foods
- Eat breakfast
- Eat foods with fiber
- Eat fruit instead of drinking fruit juice
- Choose moderate serving sizes
- Eat small amounts frequently
- Select foods that require a lot of chewing
- Eat your vegetables naked
- Prepare food without added fat
- Eat slowly
- Eat in a relaxed atmosphere
- Be aware of your body's signals

Getting Ahead Thin Habit 1: **Choose low-fat foods.** If you choose foods with less fat, your choices for the day will stretch further. For example, one tablespoon of regular stick margarine has twelve grams of fat; switch to a whipped variety and the fat drops to seven grams per tablespoon. This simple change saves five grams of fat that you can use somewhere else during the day. When you make a stir-fry dinner, coat the pan with a no-stick cooking spray (one gram of fat per spray) rather than a tablespoon of oil (fourteen grams of fat). This substitution saves thirteen grams of fat that you can enjoy some other way.

Using the Getting Ahead Menus

The Getting Ahead phase of the Fat Attack Plan lets you personalize your daily menu by adding fifteen grams of fat to a basic Menu Pattern. When you do this you'll learn which of the fat foods you regularly eat are low in fat and which of them contain more fat. At the same time, you'll be eating the right amount of fat each day to lower your cholesterol and lose weight.

On pages 164 to 219 are fourteen preplanned Getting Ahead Menu Samples followed by fourteen menu worksheets. And on pages 222 to

233 you'll find the Food Lists that will help you follow this phase of the Fat Attack Plan.

We recommend that when you begin Getting Ahead you use the fourteen preplanned menus. Each one has a breakfast, lunch, dinner, Anytime Snack, and P.M. Snack. Use one menu a day, beginning with Day 1 and going through to Day 14. Or look over the fourteen menus and pick the ones you like best. Repeat the menus you like over and over until you've followed Getting Ahead for fourteen days. Using a "28 Days to Success" calendar will help you keep track of your Getting Ahead days, particularly if you don't follow the fourteen menus in sequence.

NOW YOU TAKE OVER

Halfway through your twenty-eight days on Getting Ahead it will be time for you to take over. Instead of using preplanned menus, you'll begin designing your own daily eating plan using the Menu Worksheets.

But some of you may already be feeling very confident and eager to take charge of your Fat Attack. If that's the case, skip the fourteen preplanned menus and start Day 1 of Getting Ahead with your own personalized eating plan.

Getting Ahead, like Super Start, is very flexible. You can follow the preplanned menus for fourteen days, then take over yourself. You can follow preplanned menus on some days and customize them on others, in any order you wish. Or you can design your own menus for all twenty-eight days. It's entirely up to you!

Each Getting Ahead menu, whether planned by us or by you, is a healthy, nutritious eating plan that contains no more than fifteen grams of added Fat Choices each day. *As long as your menus don't exceed fifteen grams of added fat, it won't matter how they're put together; you'll still lose five to ten pounds, lower your cholesterol, and lower your other health risks as well.*

Just be careful to keep track of your days. It's important to stay on Getting Ahead for twenty-eight days because it takes three to four weeks of low-fat eating to make a change in your cholesterol level. (However, if you're cycling through Super Start and Getting Ahead more than once, it's okay to follow Getting Ahead for *less* than twenty-eight days the *second* time through, *if* you've reached your target weight. At that point you can move on to In Control.)

If you look over the Getting Ahead Menu Samples, you'll see a column of numbers to the right of the menu items. This is how—and where— you track your fat. The numbers represent the grams of fat added to the basic Menu Pattern. You can add fifteen grams of fat each day. In the

Getting Ahead
MENU SAMPLE—DAY 1

Menu Pattern	Today's Food Could Be	Today's Fat Grams
BREAKFAST		
1 Ounce Cereal	1 Ounce Oat Flakes	
1 Fruit Choice	2 Tablespoons Raisins	
1 Cup Skim Milk	1 Cup Skim Milk	
Coffee, Tea, or Free Drink	Tea	
*Fat Choice	*2 Tablespoons Half-and-Half	4 grams
ANYTIME SNACK		
2 Bread Choices	1 Whole Wheat Bagel	
1 Cup Skim Milk	1 Cup Skim Milk	
*Fat Choice		
LUNCH		
Free Salad	Free Salad	
1 Vegetable Choice	1 Cup Raw Zucchini Sticks	
1/2 Cup Beans or 1 Bread Choice	1/2 Cup Chick-peas	
1 Fruit Choice	1 Medium Pear	
Coffee, Tea, or Free Drink	Tea	
	*1 Ounce Lean Roast Beef	2 grams
*Fat Choice	*1 Ounce Part-skim Mozzarella Cheese	5 grams
DINNER		
1 Main Dish Choice	3 Ounces Broiled Veal Chop (Meat Only)	
1 Side Dish Choice	1 Large Baked Potato	
1 Vegetable Choice	1 Cup Cooked Mixed Vegetables	
Free Salad	Free Salad	
Coffee, Tea, or Free Drink	Coffee	
*Fat Choice	*2 Teaspoons Diet Margarine	4 grams
P.M. SNACK		
1 Fruit Choice or 4 ounces Dry or Semi-dry Wine or 2 Cups Air-popped Popcorn	1 Cup Cubed Watermelon	
	Today's Fat Choices Total	**15 grams**

* Fat choices are optional and should TOTAL no more than 15 grams of fat per day.

preplanned menus, this extra fat has been included already, but you can make different Fat Choices if you want to. That's why we've indicated an optional Fat Choice at breakfast, lunch, dinner, and the Anytime Snack. Just remember that even if you don't follow the preplanned menus, they can give you many good ideas for putting together your own low-fat meals.

The fats included in the preplanned menus come from the Fat Choices list on pages 222–23. This is a good time to take a nice long look at this list. Many of the foods on it are "visible" fats, the ones you easily recognize—butter, margarine, oil, salad dressing, and sour cream. Others have "invisible" fat. These are the foods that may not look fatty but really are—olives, nuts, cheese, and cream.

Once you move beyond the preplanned menus and begin adding your own Fat Choices to the basic Menu Pattern, write down the number of grams of fat you're adding in the column labeled "Today's Fat Choices" on the right-hand side of the Menu Worksheet. This is an easy way to keep track of the fat you're eating. Just be sure you don't add more than fifteen grams of fat per day.

On Day 1 (see the sample on page 148), two tablespoons of half-and-half (cream) are added to breakfast. This Fat Choice contains four grams of fat, so a "4" is noted in the right-hand column. That leaves eleven grams of fat to use that day.

One ounce of roast beef and one ounce of part-skim mozzarella cheese are added to lunch, totaling seven grams of fat. Subtracting four grams of fat (the breakfast Fat Choice) and seven grams of fat (the lunch Fat Choices) leaves four grams of fat to add later in the day.

At dinner, two teaspoons of diet margarine are added, using up the four remaining fat grams allowed and bringing the total fat for the day up to fifteen grams.

If you look ahead to Day 3, you'll see that fewer than fifteen grams of fat are added to the sample menu. That's fine! The key is not to exceed fifteen grams per day.

Breakfast

Getting Ahead Thin Habit 2: **Eat breakfast.** Food consumption surveys show that people who eat breakfast are thinner than breakfast skippers. There's no excuse for not giving yourself the benefit of a nutritious start to each day. Of course, you don't have to eat the second you pop out of bed. You can eat an hour later at home, or in a coffee shop on the way to work, or at work in the company cafeteria. Just don't skip this important meal with the idea that you can make up for it later in the day. Your body doesn't work that way!

CEREAL AND FRUIT: A FIBER-RICH BREAKFAST

Each Getting Ahead breakfast includes a serving of cereal, fruit, and milk, as well as coffee, tea, or a Free Drink. To this basic breakfast plan you add a Fat Choice.

One of the goals of Getting Ahead is to let you practice making good food choices. That's why you can use *any* cereal you want for breakfast —as long as it's low in fat and contains a whole-grain fiber.

Getting Ahead Thin Habit 3: **Eat foods with fiber.** A good Cereal Choice has no more than two grams of fat in a one-ounce serving, and contains fiber. The nutrition label on the side panel of the cereal box tells you how many grams of fat there are in one serving. Run your finger down the panel until you find the ingredients listing, and check to see if the cereal contains fiber. Ingredients with fiber are:

Brown rice	Oatmeal	Wheat bran
Brown-rice flour	Rice bran	Whole-kernel corn
Corn bran	Rye berries	Whole oats
Oat bran	Rye flour	Whole wheat
Oat flour	Wheat berries	Whole-wheat flour

The nutrition label on page 151 shows that Brand XXX Cereal is a good choice, with one gram of fat in a one-ounce serving and three sources of fiber: oat bran, wheat bran, and whole-wheat flour.

This cereal contains less than one gram of fat per serving and it contains three sources of fiber, which are underlined in the ingredients listing. This makes it a good choice for Getting Ahead; in fact, it's a great Cereal Choice for any phase of the Fat Attack Plan.

You can also use the Cereal Choices List on pages 224–25 to pick a breakfast cereal. All the cereals listed are low in fat and have a good amount of soluble fiber in the form of oats, oatmeal, or oat bran. As we learned in chapter 4, a diet that contains soluble fiber will help you lower both your cholesterol and your blood sugar. This is why it's so important to find a cereal high in soluble fiber for your Getting Ahead breakfast, since one of the main goals of Getting Ahead is to lower health risks, such as high blood cholesterol.

Another excellent cholesterol-lowering soluble fiber is rice bran. You get some rice bran when you eat brown rice, brown-rice flour, or cereal made from either of these. A cereal with one of these ingredients is an excellent choice on the Fat Attack Plan, provided it's also very low in fat.

Getting Ahead Thin Habit 4: **Eat fruit instead of drinking fruit juice.** Each morning, you pick a fruit for your Getting Ahead breakfast. Pick one you like from the Fruit Choices list on pages 225–26 and use it to

NUTRITION LABEL FOR A CEREAL CONTAINING FIBER

Brand XXX Cereal
NUTRITION INFORMATION

Serving Size: 1 ounce (approximately ⅔ cup)
Servings per Package: 12

	Cereal	Cereal Plus ½ Cup Skim Milk
Calories	120	160
Protein (g)	4	8
Fat (g)	1	1
Cholesterol (mg)	0	0
Sodium (mg)	220	280
Potassium (mg)	160	360

INGREDIENTS: <u>Oat bran, wheat bran, whole-wheat flour</u>, sugar, rice, corn syrup, malt flavoring, salt, baking soda.

---

top your cereal, or eat it plain. You can even save it for a midmorning snack if you want to, but be sure you eat it.

Fruit is high in fiber, and eating a piece of whole fruit rather than drinking juice will provide you with lots of chewing and the bulk that keeps your stomach fuller longer. Many fruits—such as oranges, grapefruit, and apples—also contain the soluble fiber pectin, which helps lower your cholesterol. Even better, fruits contain a wide variety of vitamins and minerals. As we learned in chapter 4, many fruits are excellent sources of vitamin A, daily doses of which are recommended by many researchers involved in cancer prevention, and several fruits are superb sources of vitamin C, which is critical to immune function.

Getting Ahead Thin Habit 5: **Choose moderate serving sizes**. The Fruit Choice portion sizes on Getting Ahead menus are ample without being excessive. Though fruits are extremely nutritious and practically fat free, it's still smart to eat moderate portions of all foods while you're trying to lose weight. When you've reached your target weight, you can have larger portions of fruit if you'd like to.

A cup of skim milk is planned for breakfast. Use it on your cereal, as a drink, or in your coffee or tea. Skim milk contains very little fat, and is a wonderful source of calcium. In fact, the milk you have with your Getting Ahead breakfast provides more than one-third of your daily calcium needs.

You can have a Free Drink at breakfast, too. Choose from the Free Drinks on page 232 for beverages to have at various times throughout the day. These are "free," so you can have as much as you want. They'll fill you up and keep you satisfied; moreover, plenty of liquid is essential to your body if it is to function properly. Five drinks are planned for each day on the Getting Ahead menus, but since nutrition experts recommend six to eight cups of liquid each day, do add several more Free Drinks throughout the day.

Just be sure to keep your coffee and tea consumption low; they're not *Free* Drinks. Caffeine can make you jumpy and grouchy, and coffee, whether regular or decaffeinated, has even been shown to raise cholesterol levels.

AND HERE'S THE BEST PART

You still have the option of adding a Fat Choice at breakfast, which will become part of the fifteen grams of fat you'll add throughout the day. Fat Choices are listed on pages 222–23. You may want a little cream in your tea, an egg, a piece of cheese, or any other fat food from the list. The grams of fat from the Fat Choice should be listed in the right-hand column on the Menu Worksheet.

Your Anytime Snack

The Anytime Snack is just that—a snack you can have at any point during the day. Because a midmorning coffee break is very typical in this country, we've placed the snack midmorning on your Menu Pattern. But you certainly don't have to eat it then! Many of our clients, particularly the ones who commute a long distance to work and eat a late dinner, enjoy this snack in the mid- to late afternoon.

Getting Ahead Thin Habit 6: **Eat small amounts frequently**. Have this snack whenever you wish. You don't even have to eat the whole thing all at once. But it *is* important to snack—on the right foods at the right times. When should you snack? When you feel hungry, when you feel you *want* your snack, not just when the clock says it's time to snack.

We've learned from research that snackers are leaner than nonsnackers. And nutrition experts at the International Diabetes Center in Minnesota recommend snacking to prevent wide fluctuations in blood glucose (sugar). They also suggest eating between-meal snacks to control appetite, which in turn makes weight loss easier. So don't worry that snacking will do your diet in. The right snack will do just the reverse!

A MINI-MEAL

The Anytime Snack includes two Bread Choices from the list on page 227 and another cup of skim milk. This is a good time to think about adding a Fat Choice, possibly a slice of cheese, to create a snack that's almost a meal. Depending on your schedule, this could be a real boon to your diet by providing a filling pick-me-up either in the middle of a morning or on the long train ride home from work.

The second cup of milk is built into the snack to meet your adult requirement for two servings of milk each day. But you don't have to have it all with your snack; you could use some for tea in the afternoon and save the rest for dinner. Do drink it, though, to ensure that you get adequate calcium and other vital nutrients, like vitamin D.

UNDERSTANDING YOUR BREAD CHOICES

One Bread Choice (see the list on page 227) generally equals one slice of bread, but there are a few exceptions. For example, half a bagel equals one Bread Choice (or, one bagel equals two Bread Choices). Since the Anytime Snack has two Bread Choices, you could have a whole bagel at snack time. The same two-for-one rule applies to many other Bread Choices as well: A hamburger bun, a hot-dog roll, and a hard roll are equal to two Bread Choices each. Just think of one slice of bread as being equal to half a roll.

But one slice or two, not all Bread Choices are the same where fat is concerned. A few choices, such as brown bread, cinnamon bread, and raisin bread, allow you only *half* a slice for one Bread Choice. That's because these choices are a little more cakelike and contain more fat, so the serving size has to be smaller.

In Getting Ahead you'll be making many food choices on your own. Deciding to have raisin bread as a snack with the realization that you can have only one slice is a good example of how you'll learn to make sensible fat-food choices. Another sensible Bread Choice to make whenever possible is whole-grain bread. This type of bread has more of the original fiber and offers you all the nutritional benefits of unrefined grain.

MAKE A FAT CHOICE

You can top your bread or bagel with jam, jelly, or any other Getting Ahead Free Sweet (see the list on page 233). Or you can use a Fat Choice. Cream cheese, margarine, cottage cheese, and butter are all possibilities. Drizzle one tablespoon of reduced-calorie Italian dressing on Italian bread and sprinkle it with garlic powder (it's "free"). Pop it in the micro-wave for about 20 seconds, or under the broiler until it's golden brown. You've used up only two grams of fat for a great snack.

One ounce of cheddar cheese melted on top of an English muffin is another satisfying snack, with nine grams of fat. You could even make a quick bagel pizza by topping bagel halves with sliced tomatoes ("free," from the Salad Fixings list on page 232), one ounce of grated part-skim mozzarella cheese, some oregano ("free"), and a sliced large black olive. Add up the fat grams: five for the cheese and two for the olive make seven. If these were your first fat grams for the day, you'd still have eight more to go. That's a lot of very tasty additions to your daily Getting Ahead menu—and you'd still be losing weight.

Lunch

Now that you've finished snacking, it's time for lunch! Each Getting Ahead lunch includes a Free Salad, one Vegetable Choice, a half-cup of beans or one Bread Choice, one Fruit Choice, and coffee, tea, or a Free Drink. You can also add any Fat Choice you wish.

FREE SALAD

Getting Ahead Thin Habit 7: **Select foods that require a lot of chewing**. At lunch you get to invent a different Free Salad every day using Free Salad Fixings (page 232). You decide what to use and how big you want your salad to be. Salad Fixings are "free" foods because they're virtually fat free—so have as much as you want. They're also rich in vitamins, minerals, and fiber; they'll keep you chewing during your meal—and satisfied after it.

You may enjoy your Free Salad plain, or you can use a dash of flavored vinegar, some lemon or lime juice, one of the Free Condiments from the list on page 233, our own "Zero Dressing" (see the recipe on page 78), or a no-oil dressing that you buy at the market. The no-oil dressing should be just that: It should show "0 grams" of fat on the nutrition label.

This may also be a good time to add a Fat Choice. There are a number of salad dressings to choose from on the Fat Choices list. Or, one table-spoon of olive oil will give your salad a flavor lift. It adds fifteen grams of fat, but if that's what you'd like, go ahead. This kind of freedom is what makes Getting Ahead such a wonderful eating plan.

PICK YOUR VEGETABLE

There are dozens to choose from on the Vegetable Choices list on page 228. Once you've picked it, you can decide if you'd like to have it cooked or raw. It can be used as a side dish or vegetable choice, or incorporated into your Free Salad.

Getting Ahead Thin Habit 8: **Eat your vegetables naked**. Vegetables are rich in vitamins, minerals, and fiber, and most are very low in fat. You should probably keep yours that way, unless you decide to use one of your fat choices to "dress" them.

BREAD OR BEANS?

Decide if you want one Bread Choice or a half-cup of beans at lunch. They're similar in that they're both low in fat and high in fiber. Since you're having bread for your Anytime Snack, a nice change for lunch is to have the beans instead. You can have just about any kind of beans you'd like; they come in an endless array. There are chick-peas, lima beans, kidney beans, white beans, and black-eyed peas, to name a few. They're low in fat and high in soluble fiber. They're vitamin- and mineral-rich, and they fill you up nicely.

Buy them canned, or cook them yourself right from the bag. Just be aware that this takes quite a bit of time. If you decide to start with dried beans, we recommend that you cook a whole one-pound bag and freeze the beans in half-cup portions. Storing them in resealable plastic bags makes it easy to defrost them in the microwave.

You can combine them with your Vegetable Choice or put them in your Free Salad. Or you can turn them into a salad by adding vinegar, salsa, a Free Condiment from the list on page 233, or even a little oil if you'd like to use some of your fat grams. Eaten hot, all varieties of beans can be flavored quickly with chopped onions, green onions, peppers, tomatoes, or any of the other Free Salad Fixings on page 232, which you can also sauté first in a little cooking spray if you want to.

TOP OFF YOUR MEAL WITH FRUIT

Select a Fruit Choice (see the list on pages 225–26) and have it as part of lunch, or as a snack you save for later. You can even take an apple or a pear and bake it in the microwave with some cinnamon for a cozy midafternoon pick-me-up.

Like all the other meals in your Getting Ahead Menu Pattern, lunch has endless possibilities. The menu pattern for lunch can easily be fulfilled with selections from a salad bar or at a restaurant featuring fresh salads. Or you may want to use the Bread Choice plus a Fat Choice to make an open-faced sandwich. The Getting Ahead Menu Samples on pages 165–91 offer many interesting ideas for creative meals using your basic Menu Pattern and your fat allowance. Use the menu samples to tickle your own imagination; we know you can come up with a lot more!

And don't forget to *keep track of your Fat Choices* by writing them down in the right-hand column of your Getting Ahead Menu Worksheet. All of us have favorite foods that we pick frequently; you'll begin to see which of your favorites contain fat and how much fat there is in the serving you usually have. By keeping track of the fat you add to your meals during Getting Ahead, you'll be setting the stage for taking control of *all* your food choices when you move into In Control at the end of your twenty-eight days.

Dinner

Each Getting Ahead dinner has a Free Salad, one Main Dish, one Side Dish, one Vegetable Choice, and coffee, tea, or a Free Drink. You can add any Fat Choice you wish.

Pick your Main Dish from the choices on pages 228–30—and be sure to use the portion size recommended. All portion sizes are given in ounces and refer to the weight of the meat only, after cooking. The weight doesn't include fat or bone. When you buy boneless meat, fish, or poultry, choose a piece that's about one ounce heavier than the recommended portion size; you'll lose that ounce in the cooking process. When you buy bone-in meat or poultry, a five-ounce raw piece will give you a three-ounce edible cooked portion.

You're probably wondering why all the serving sizes on the list aren't the same. It's simply because all protein foods don't contain the same amount of fat. Some have more, like certain cuts of pork and beef; some have less, like many fish. Using the recommended portion sizes ensures that the amount of fat you eat will be approximately the same, no matter what choice you make. Right now you don't have to keep track of the fat in the Main Dishes you choose, but it helps to understand why the serving sizes vary. All the things you learn in Getting Ahead will help you later, when you're In Control, particularly when you're making selections from foods that can contain a large amount of fat.

Getting Ahead Thin Habit 9: **Prepare food without added fat**. Prepare your choice by grilling, broiling, steaming, baking, roasting, poaching, or stir-frying. To add flavor, use Free Salad Fixings, Free Condiments, and Free Sweets when preparing your food for cooking, or add them at the table. In Super Start, you learned to prepare your Main Dish foods with no added fat at all. The cooking tips you learned are good ones to remember through Getting Ahead and right into In Control.

Or you can use your Fat Choice to prepare or top off your Main Dish. Just be careful—be sure to count all the added fat into the day's total. You can't add more than fifteen grams of fat each day!

YOUR SIDE DISH

Along with your Main Dish, each dinner has a Side Dish. Make your choice from the list of Side Dish Choices, which you'll find on pages 230–32. And be sure to use the recommended serving size. There are many good recipe ideas for interesting side dishes in Super Start on pages 78–132. Boiled, baked, or steamed, all the choices are virtually fat free. But now that you're in Getting Ahead, you may want to add a Fat Choice to one of these Side Dishes. Just be sure to track the fat.

Noodles aren't included on the list because most are made with eggs and therefore contain some fat. But if you can find "no-egg" or "no-egg-yolk" noodles at your supermarket, they'd be fine for a Getting Ahead Side Dish.

VEGETABLES IN ALL FORMS

Next, plan one vegetable from the Vegetable Choices list on page 228. Vegetables add flavor, color, texture, fiber, and nutrients to a meal. Use a wide variety and enjoy them! There are so many on the list, there's a good chance there are many you've never even eaten. So give a few new ones a try. Eat them plain tonight to see how they really taste (and to save your Fat Choices), and then decide if you'd like to have them cooked or raw in your salad tomorrow night.

Just be sure you have the recommended portion size. Although vegetables are rich in nutrients and fiber and are virtually fat free, it's important while you're losing weight to eat moderate servings. Later, when you're In Control, you can have extra servings of vegetables, if you'd like, because then they'll qualify as "free" foods.

DON'T FORGET YOUR SALAD!

Every Getting Ahead dinner includes a salad as large as you'd like; you can pick from the dozens of Free Salad Fixings on page 232 to create a colorful, crunchy bowlful. Fresh, lush salads are a dieting plus. They offer great nutritional value, no fat, lots of fiber, and the satisfaction of chewing. If you still have Fat Choice grams left for the day, you may want to "splurge" with a dressing from the Fat Choices list (page 223) to top your salad. Otherwise, enjoy a no-oil dressing or Zero Dressing (see page 78), or perhaps something from the Free Condiments list on page 233.

TO CONCLUDE YOUR MEAL

Pour your coffee, tea, or Free Drink and take a few moments to think about some other things. Was this evening's dinner a relaxed, pleasant meal—or was it a quickie that gave you indigestion because you bolted it down too fast?

Getting Ahead Thin Habits 10 and 11: **Eat slowly. Eat in a relaxed atmosphere**. For many people, dinner is the first time during the day that they really get to slow down and catch their breath. Many of us don't even see our families until we get home for dinner. So make it a pleasant one. Plan to eat in a comfortable, relaxed atmosphere. Even if you normally eat alone, treat yourself like company. Buy some flowers, play some music, and set the stage for a lovely meal. Where and how you eat are almost as important as what you eat. Be good to yourself!

A SNACK TO END THE DAY

Your P.M. Snack doesn't have to actually end the day, but it's nice to know you can have something more before bedtime. Have it any time you wish after dinner. It can be your dessert, or you can sit up in bed with a book and the snack of your choice.

Choose whatever you wish to snack on: one fruit from the Fruit Choices list (pages 225–26), four ounces of dry or semi-dry wine, or two cups of air-popped popcorn. All of these are virtually fat free, and any one of them would be a nice way to end the day. Just eat, or drink, your snack slowly. In fact, it's a good idea to take a full ten minutes to finish your snack.

Getting Ahead Thin Habit 12: **Be aware of your body's signals**. After your P.M. Snack, sit back and think about how satisfied you feel. As silly as it sounds, it takes time for your brain to get the message that you've been fed. But being in tune with your body is one of the best ways to stay on track—and to Get Ahead.

Your Twenty-Eight Days Are Up!

As you plan your Menu Worksheet each day, choosing foods and keeping track of Fat Choices, you'll become increasingly aware of those foods that contain fat. You'll make better and better Fat Choices and you'll come closer to your target weight and health goals. And before you know it, you'll be finished.

If you've completed both Super Start and Getting Ahead, you've lost twenty-five pounds and significantly lowered your cholesterol and other health risks. Terrific! Move on to In Control. You're ready to take charge.

If you started the Fat Attack Plan with Getting Ahead, you've lost five to ten pounds and your cholesterol has dropped significantly. You're doing great! You're ready to be In Control, too.

If your target weight loss was more than twenty-five pounds, you need to work on losing weight for a little while longer. By now you've seen a substantial weight loss, so you're confident the Fat Attack Plan works. Let it continue to work for you! If your target weight is more than fifteen pounds away, cycle back to Super Start for a second twenty-eight days, then use Getting Ahead for a second time. If your target weight is just ten pounds away, or less, simply stay on Getting Ahead for a second twenty-eight days. Then, as soon as you reach your target weight, move on to In Control.

Just remember—twenty-eight days goes very fast when you're following a plan as good as the Fat Attack Plan. The rewards of weight loss, better health, longer life, and the freedom of being In Control can all be yours—just for the Super Starting and Getting Ahead. Good luck!

Getting Ahead
MENUS AND
WORKSHEETS

On the following pages you'll find fourteen days of Getting Ahead Menu Samples. They're good illustrations of the kinds of foods you can work into your new low-fat eating plan.

As you start Getting Ahead, we recommend that you follow these menus for your first fourteen days. Look them over and pick the ones you like best; you can repeat them as often as you'd like, if that's what you want to do.

If you don't like one of the Fat Choices we've suggested on a given day, you don't need to eat it. In fact, you can replace it with another Fat Choice of your own sometime during the day. Just be sure the Fat Choice you make doesn't bring your total fat count for the day over fifteen grams.

Then you'll see Menu Worksheets for Days 15–28. Beginning with Day 15, you fill in all the blanks with the foods of your choice.

Be sure to track your fat. Now you're Getting Ahead!

Getting Ahead
MENU PATTERN

BREAKFAST
Cereal Choice
Fruit Choice
Skim Milk
Coffee, Tea, or Free Drink
Fat Choice

ANYTIME SNACK
2 Bread Choices
Skim Milk
Fat Choice

LUNCH
Free Salad
Vegetable Choice
Beans or Bread Choice
Fruit Choice
Coffee, Tea, or Free Drink
Fat Choice

DINNER
Main Dish Choice
Side Dish Choice
Vegetable Choice
Free Salad
Coffee, Tea, or Free Drink
Fat Choice

** Fat choices are
optional and
should TOTAL no
more than 15 grams
of fat per day.*

P.M. SNACK
*Fruit Choice or
Dry or Semi-dry Wine or
Air-popped Popcorn*

Personalizing the *Getting Ahead* MENU PATTERN

The Getting Ahead Menu Pattern offers so many choices that designing your meals is almost entirely up to you. You'll find there's a lot of choice built into the 14 days of preplanned menus we offer to get you started. Or, if you wish, you can begin putting your own meals together from Day 1. Whichever way you do it, for each underlined menu item below refer to the Food List on the page indicated to make your choice.

BREAKFAST
Cereal Choice (pages 224–25)
Fruit Choice (pages 225–26)
Skim Milk
Coffee, Tea, or Free Drink (page 232)
*Fat Choice (pages 222–23)

ANYTIME SNACK
2 Bread Choices (page 227)
Skim Milk
*Fat Choice (pages 222–23)

LUNCH
Free Salad (page 232)
Vegetable Choice (page 228)
Beans or Bread Choice (page 227)
Fruit Choice (pages 225–26)
Coffee, Tea, or Free Drink (page 232)
*Fat Choice (pages 222–23)

DINNER
Main Dish Choice (pages 228–30)
Side Dish Choice (pages 230–32)
Vegetable Choice (page 228)
Free Salad (page 232)
Coffee, Tea, or Free Drink (page 232)
*Fat Choice (pages 222–23)

* Fat choices are optional and should TOTAL no more than 15 grams of fat per day.

P.M. SNACK
Fruit Choice (pages 225–26) or Wine or Popcorn

Getting Ahead
MENU SAMPLE—DAY 1

Menu Pattern

BREAKFAST
1 Ounce Cereal Choice
1 Fruit Choice
1 Cup Skim Milk
Coffee, Tea, or Free Drink
***Fat Choice**

ANYTIME SNACK
2 Bread Choices
1 Cup Skim Milk
***Fat Choice**

LUNCH
Free Salad
1 Vegetable Choice
¹/₂ Cup Beans **or** *1 Bread Choice*
1 Fruit Choice
Coffee, Tea, or Free Drink
***Fat Choice**

DINNER
1 Main Dish Choice
1 Side Dish Choice
1 Vegetable Choice
Free Salad
Coffee, Tea, or Free Drink
***Fat Choice**

*** Fat choices are optional and should TOTAL no more than 15 grams of fat per day.**

P.M. SNACK
1 Fruit Choice **or**
4 Ounces Dry **or** *Semi-dry Wine* **or**
2 Cups Air-popped Popcorn

Today's Food Could Be	Today's Fat Grams

BREAKFAST

1 oz oat flakes

2 tbsp raisins

1 cup skim milk

tea

* 2 tbsp half-and-half   4

ANYTIME SNACK

1 whole wheat bagel

1 cup skim milk

*

LUNCH

Free Salad

1 cup raw zucchini sticks

½ cup chick-peas

1 medium pear

tea

* 1 oz lean roast beef   2

* 1 oz part-skim mozzarella cheese   5

DINNER

3 oz broiled veal chop (meat only)

1 large baked potato

1 cup cooked mixed vegetables

Free Salad

coffee

* 2 tsp diet margarine   4

P.M. SNACK

1 cup cubed watermelon

Today's Fat Choices Total   15

Getting Ahead
MENU SAMPLE—DAY 2

Menu Pattern

BREAKFAST
1 Ounce Cereal Choice
1 Fruit Choice
1 Cup Skim Milk
Coffee, Tea, or Free Drink
***Fat Choice**

ANYTIME SNACK
2 Bread Choices
1 Cup Skim Milk
***Fat Choice**

LUNCH
Free Salad
1 Vegetable Choice
½ Cup Beans or 1 Bread Choice
1 Fruit Choice
Coffee, Tea, or Free Drink
***Fat Choice**

DINNER
1 Main Dish Choice
1 Side Dish Choice
1 Vegetable Choice
Free Salad
Coffee, Tea, or Free Drink
***Fat Choice**

*** Fat choices are optional and should TOTAL no more than 15 grams of fat per day.**

P.M. SNACK
1 Fruit Choice or
4 Ounces Dry or Semi-dry Wine or
2 Cups Air-popped Popcorn

Today's Food Could Be	*Today's Fat Grams*

BREAKFAST
1 oz Bite-size Shredded Wheat
1 small banana
1 cup skim milk
coffee
*_____   _____

ANYTIME SNACK
1 raisin bagel
1 cup skim milk
* 1 oz whipped cream cheese   10

LUNCH
Free Salad
1 cup raw carrot sticks
1 slice pumpernickel bread
1 small bunch grapes
mineral water
* ½ cup 1% cottage cheese   1

DINNER
5 oz steamed shrimp
3/4 cup cooked rice
1 cup broccoli
Free Salad
iced tea
* 2 tbsp reduced-calorie Italian dressing   4

P.M. SNACK
8 dried apricot halves

                    Today's Fat Choices Total   15

Getting Ahead
MENU SAMPLE—DAY 3
BUSINESS LUNCH DAY

Menu Pattern

BREAKFAST
1 Ounce Cereal Choice
1 Fruit Choice
1 Cup Skim Milk
Coffee, Tea, or Free Drink
*Fat Choice

ANYTIME SNACK
2 Bread Choices
1 Cup Skim Milk
*Fat Choice

†LUNCH
1 Main Dish Choice
1 Side Dish Choice
1 Vegetable Choice
Free Salad
Coffee, Tea, or Free Drink
*Fat Choice

†DINNER
Free Salad
1 Vegetable Choice
1/2 Cup Beans or 1 Bread Choice
1 Fruit Choice
Coffee, Tea, or Free Drink
*Fat Choice

P.M. SNACK
1 Fruit Choice or
4 Ounces Dry or Semi-dry Wine or
2 Cups Air-popped Popcorn

* *Fat choices are optional and should TOTAL no more than 15 grams of fat per day.*

† *On a day when you have a business lunch scheduled, simply switch lunch and dinner.*

168 · *Getting Ahead*

Today's Food Could Be	Today's Fat Grams

Today's Food Could Be

Today's Fat Grams

BREAKFAST
1 oz puffed rice

1 large orange

1 cup skim milk

tea

* _____

ANYTIME SNACK
2 slices rye toast

1 cup skim milk

* _____

LUNCH
½ roasted chicken breast (no skin)

½ cup cooked lentils

1 cup steamed asparagus

Free Salad

tea

* 1 tbsp blue cheese dressing   8

DINNER
Free Salad

1 cup raw cauliflower

1 slice whole wheat bread

1 kiwi

mineral water

* 2 oz tuna (canned in water)   1

* 1 tbsp reduced-calorie mayonnaise   5

P.M. SNACK
4 oz wine

Today's Fat Choices Total   14

Getting Ahead
MENU SAMPLE—DAY 4

Menu Pattern

BREAKFAST
1 Ounce Cereal Choice
1 Fruit Choice
1 Cup Skim Milk
Coffee, Tea, or Free Drink
***Fat Choice**

ANYTIME SNACK
2 Bread Choices
1 Cup Skim Milk
***Fat Choice**

LUNCH
Free Salad
1 Vegetable Choice
½ Cup Beans or 1 Bread Choice
1 Fruit Choice
Coffee, Tea, or Free Drink
***Fat Choice**

DINNER
1 Main Dish Choice
1 Side Dish Choice
1 Vegetable Choice
Free Salad
Coffee, Tea, or Free Drink
***Fat Choice**

* *Fat choices are optional and should TOTAL no more than 15 grams of fat per day.*

P.M. SNACK
1 Fruit Choice or
4 Ounces Dry or Semi-dry Wine or
2 Cups Air-popped Popcorn

Today's Food Could Be	Today's Fat Grams

BREAKFAST
1 oz Raisin Bran
1 medium grapefruit
1 cup skim milk
Postum
* 2 tbsp half-and-half   4

ANYTIME SNACK
2 slices rye bread
1 cup skim milk
*

LUNCH
Free Salad
1 cup raw carrot sticks
½ cup cooked red kidney beans
2 plums
lemon/lime seltzer
* ¼ avocado   7

DINNER
3 oz broiled ground round patty
3/4 cup cooked elbow macaroni
1 cup baked acorn squash
Free Salad
herb tea
* 1 tbsp grated Parmesan cheese   2
* 1 tbsp reduced-calorie Italian dressing   2

P.M. SNACK
1 small bunch grapes

Today's Fat Choices Total   15

Getting Ahead
MENU SAMPLE—DAY 5

Menu Pattern

BREAKFAST
1 Ounce Cereal Choice
1 Fruit Choice
1 Cup Skim Milk
Coffee, Tea, or Free Drink
*Fat Choice

ANYTIME SNACK
2 Bread Choices
1 Cup Skim Milk
*Fat Choice

LUNCH
Free Salad
1 Vegetable Choice
½ Cup Beans or 1 Bread Choice
1 Fruit Choice
Coffee, Tea, or Free Drink
*Fat Choice

DINNER
1 Main Dish Choice
1 Side Dish Choice
1 Vegetable Choice
Free Salad
Coffee, Tea, or Free Drink
*Fat Choice

* Fat choices are optional and should TOTAL no more than 15 grams of fat per day.

P.M. SNACK
1 Fruit Choice or
4 Ounces Dry or Semi-dry Wine or
2 Cups Air-popped Popcorn

Today's Food
Could Be

BREAKFAST
1 oz All Bran
1 large nectarine
1 cup skim milk
coffee
*

ANYTIME SNACK
1 plain bagel
1 cup skim milk
* 1 tbsp peanut butter   8

LUNCH
Free salad
1 medium apple
iced tea
1 cup cooked sliced beets (chilled)
Open-faced "BLT": 1 slice toast
*   2 tsp reduced-calorie mayonnaise   4
*   1 strip cooked bacon   3

DINNER
4 oz roasted turkey breast (no skin)
3/4 cup steamed brown rice
1 cup steamed sugar snap peas
Free salad
herb tea
*

P.M. SNACK
4 oz wine

                    Today's Fat Choices Total   15

Getting Ahead
MENU SAMPLE—DAY 6

Menu Pattern

BREAKFAST
1 Ounce Cereal Choice
1 Fruit Choice
1 Cup Skim Milk
Coffee, Tea, or Free Drink
Fat Choice

ANYTIME SNACK
2 Bread Choices
1 Cup Skim Milk
Fat Choice

LUNCH
Free Salad
1 Vegetable Choice
½ Cup Beans or 1 Bread Choice
1 Fruit Choice
Coffee, Tea, or Free Drink
Fat Choice

DINNER
1 Main Dish Choice
1 Side Dish Choice
1 Vegetable Choice
Free Salad
Coffee, Tea, or Free Drink
Fat Choice

P.M. SNACK
1 Fruit Choice or
4 Ounces Dry or Semi-dry Wine or
2 Cups Air-popped Popcorn

* Fat choices are optional and should TOTAL no more than 15 grams of fat per day.

Today's Food
Could Be

Today's
Fat Grams

BREAKFAST
1 oz oat flakes
1 large peach
1 cup skim milk
coffee
* _____   _____

ANYTIME SNACK
1 whole wheat English muffin
1 cup skim milk
* _____   _____

LUNCH
Free Salad
1 cup raw yellow squash
1 slice pumpernickel bread
1 medium pear
tea
* 1 hard-cooked egg   6

DINNER
3 oz broiled salmon fillet
1 large baked potato
1 cup steamed broccoli
Free Salad
mineral water
* 3 tbsp reduced-calorie French dressing   3
* 1 oz feta cheese   6

P.M. SNACK
½ mango

Today's Fat Choices Total   15

GETTING AHEAD MENUS AND WORKSHEETS · 175

Getting Ahead
MENU SAMPLE—DAY 7

Menu Pattern

BREAKFAST
1 Ounce Cereal Choice
1 Fruit Choice
1 Cup Skim Milk
Coffee, Tea, or Free Drink
*Fat Choice

ANYTIME SNACK
2 Bread Choices
1 Cup Skim Milk
*Fat Choice

LUNCH
Free Salad
1 Vegetable Choice
1/2 Cup Beans or 1 Bread Choice
1 Fruit Choice
Coffee, Tea, or Free Drink
*Fat Choice

DINNER
1 Main Dish Choice
1 Side Dish Choice
1 Vegetable Choice
Free Salad
Coffee, Tea, or Free Drink
*Fat Choice

* Fat choices are optional and should TOTAL no more than 15 grams of fat per day.

P.M. SNACK
1 Fruit Choice or
4 Ounces Dry or Semi-dry Wine or
2 Cups Air-popped Popcorn

Today's Food Could Be	Today's Fat Grams

BREAKFAST
1 oz hot wheat cereal
2 tangerines
1 cup skim milk
Pero
*

ANYTIME SNACK
1 poppy seed bagel
1 cup skim milk
* 1 oz reduced-fat cream cheese — 5

LUNCH
Free Salad
1 cup raw zucchini sticks
2 breadsticks
½ cup canned pineapple
diet cola
* 1 oz lean ham — 3

DINNER
3 oz broiled flank steak
¾ cup mashed potatoes
1 cup steamed green beans
Free Salad
coffee
* 1 tsp butter — 4
* 3 tbsp reduced-calorie French dressing — 3

P.M. SNACK
15 cherries

Today's Fat Choices Total — 15 .

Getting Ahead
MENU SAMPLE—DAY 8

Menu Pattern

BREAKFAST
1 Ounce Cereal Choice
1 Fruit Choice
1 Cup Skim Milk
Coffee, Tea, or Free Drink
***Fat Choice**

ANYTIME SNACK
2 Bread Choices
1 Cup Skim Milk
***Fat Choice**

LUNCH
Free Salad
1 Vegetable Choice
½ Cup Beans or 1 Bread Choice
1 Fruit Choice
Coffee, Tea, or Free Drink
***Fat Choice**

DINNER
1 Main Dish Choice
1 Side Dish Choice
1 Vegetable Choice
Free Salad
Coffee, Tea, or Free Drink
***Fat Choice**

P.M. SNACK
1 Fruit Choice or
4 Ounces Dry or Semi-dry Wine or
2 Cups Air-popped Popcorn

***Fat choices are
optional and
should TOTAL no
more than 15 grams
of fat per day.**

*Today's Food
Could Be*

*Today's
Fat Grams*

BREAKFAST
1 oz Shredded Wheat
1/8 honeydew melon
1 cup skim milk
coffee
*_____

ANYTIME SNACK
2 slices whole wheat bread
1 cup skim milk
*_____

LUNCH
Free Salad
1 cup sliced raw jicama
1/2 cup black-eyed peas
1 large nectarine
tea
* 1 oz cubed mozzarella cheese   6
* 1 tbsp reduced-calorie Italian dressing   2

DINNER
6 oz grilled flounder fillet
3/4 cup steamed rice
1 cup mashed turnips
Free Salad
diet ginger ale
* 3 large black olives   6

P.M. SNACK
4 oz wine

                Today's Fat Choices Total   14

Getting Ahead
MENU SAMPLE—DAY 9

Menu Pattern

BREAKFAST
1 Ounce Cereal Choice
1 Fruit Choice
1 Cup Skim Milk
Coffee, Tea, or Free Drink
Fat Choice

ANYTIME SNACK
2 Bread Choices
1 Cup Skim Milk
Fat Choice

LUNCH
Free Salad
1 Vegetable Choice
½ Cup Beans or 1 Bread Choice
1 Fruit Choice
Coffee, Tea, or Free Drink
Fat Choice

DINNER
1 Main Dish Choice
1 Side Dish Choice
1 Vegetable Choice
Free Salad
Coffee, Tea, or Free Drink
Fat Choice

P.M. SNACK
1 Fruit Choice or
4 Ounces Dry or Semi-dry Wine or
2 Cups Air-popped Popcorn

** Fat choices are
optional and
should TOTAL no
more than 15 grams
of fat per day.*

Today's Food Could Be	Today's Fat Grams

BREAKFAST
1 oz cornflakes
1 medium baked apple
1 cup skim milk
decaffeinated coffee
*

ANYTIME SNACK
1 whole wheat bagel
1 cup skim milk
*

LUNCH
Free Salad
1 cup steamed wax beans
1 medium persimmon
diet orange soda
grilled open-faced sandwich: 1 slice rye
*   1 oz Swiss cheese   8
*   1 oz lean ham   3

DINNER
3 oz roasted boneless leg of lamb
1 medium baked sweet potato
1 cup steamed corn
Free Salad
coffee
* 4 tbsp reduced-calorie French dressing   4

P.M. SNACK
2 cups air-popped popcorn

Today's Fat Choices Total   15

Getting Ahead
MENU SAMPLE—DAY 10

Menu Pattern

BREAKFAST
1 Ounce Cereal Choice
1 Fruit Choice
1 Cup Skim Milk
Coffee, Tea, or Free Drink
Fat Choice

ANYTIME SNACK
2 Bread Choices
1 Cup Skim Milk
Fat Choice

LUNCH
Free Salad
1 Vegetable Choice
½ Cup Beans or 1 Bread Choice
1 Fruit Choice
Coffee, Tea, or Free Drink
Fat Choice

DINNER
1 Main Dish Choice
1 Side Dish Choice
1 Vegetable Choice
Free Salad
Coffee, Tea, or Free Drink
Fat Choice

* Fat choices are optional and should TOTAL no more than 15 grams of fat per day.

P.M. SNACK
1 Fruit Choice or
4 Ounces Dry or Semi-dry Wine or
2 Cups Air-popped Popcorn

Today's Food Could Be	Today's Fat Grams

BREAKFAST

1 oz oatmeal

4 small apricots

1 cup skim milk

decaffeinated coffee

* _____ _____

ANYTIME SNACK

1 hard roll

1 cup skim milk

* 1 tbsp whipped butter   9

LUNCH

Free Salad

1 cup raw broccoli

1 slice pumpernickel bread

1 large peach

mineral water

* ½ cup 2% cottage cheese   4

DINNER

stir fry: ½ cup raw pea pods

   ½ cup sliced raw zucchini

   5 oz raw boneless chicken breast

¾ cup steamed brown rice

Free Salad

tea

* cooking spray   2

P.M. SNACK

1 cup raspberries

Today's Fat Choices Total   15

Getting Ahead
MENU SAMPLE—DAY 11

Menu Pattern

BREAKFAST
1 Ounce Cereal Choice
1 Fruit Choice
1 Cup Skim Milk
Coffee, Tea, or Free Drink
***Fat Choice**

ANYTIME SNACK
2 Bread Choices
1 Cup Skim Milk
***Fat Choice**

LUNCH
Free Salad
1 Vegetable Choice
½ Cup Beans or 1 Bread Choice
1 Fruit Choice
Coffee, Tea, or Free Drink
***Fat Choice**

DINNER
1 Main Dish Choice
1 Side Dish Choice
1 Vegetable Choice
Free Salad
Coffee, Tea, or Free Drink
***Fat Choice**

P.M. SNACK
1 Fruit Choice or
4 Ounces Dry or Semi-dry Wine or
2 Cups Air-popped Popcorn

*** Fat choices are
optional and
should TOTAL no
more than 15 grams
of fat per day.**

Today's Food Could Be	Today's Fat Grams

BREAKFAST

1 oz wheat flakes

1½ cups strawberries

1 cup skim milk

coffee

* _____ _____

ANYTIME SNACK

1 English muffin

1 cup skim milk

* _____ _____

LUNCH

Free Salad

1 cup raw cauliflower

1 slice whole wheat bread

2 plums

orange-flavored seltzer

* 2 oz tuna (canned in water)   1

DINNER

3 oz broiled beef tenderloin fillet

¾ cup tricolor pasta

1 cup steamed Brussels sprouts

Free Salad

tea

* 1 oz peanuts   14

P.M. SNACK

1 small banana

Today's Fat Choices Total   15

Getting Ahead
MENU SAMPLE—DAY 12

Menu Pattern

BREAKFAST
1 Ounce Cereal Choice
1 Fruit Choice
1 Cup Skim Milk
Coffee, Tea, or Free Drink
*Fat Choice

ANYTIME SNACK
2 Bread Choices
1 Cup Skim Milk
*Fat Choice

LUNCH
Free Salad
1 Vegetable Choice
½ Cup Beans or 1 Bread Choice
1 Fruit Choice
Coffee, Tea, or Free Drink
*Fat Choice

DINNER
1 Main Dish Choice
1 Side Dish Choice
1 Vegetable Choice
Free Salad
Coffee, Tea, or Free Drink
*Fat Choice

* *Fat choices are optional and should TOTAL no more than 15 grams of fat per day.*

P.M. SNACK
1 Fruit Choice or
4 Ounces Dry or Semi-dry Wine or
2 Cups Air-popped Popcorn

Today's Food Could Be	Today's Fat Grams

BREAKFAST
1 oz Raisin Bran
1 cup blueberries
1 cup skim milk
coffee
*_____

ANYTIME SNACK
1 slice brown bread
1 cup skim milk
*_____

LUNCH
Free Salad
1 cup steamed artichoke hearts (chilled)
1 slice rye bread
1/4 medium cantaloupe
diet cola
* 1 oz Muenster cheese   9
* 1 hard-cooked egg   6

DINNER
1 chicken leg + thigh (no skin)
1 cup parslied potatoes
1 cup steamed asparagus tips
Free Salad
mineral water
*_____

P.M. SNACK
1 cup cubed watermelon

Today's Fat Choices Total   15

Getting Ahead
MENU SAMPLE—DAY 13

Menu Pattern

BREAKFAST
1 Ounce Cereal Choice
1 Fruit Choice
1 Cup Skim Milk
Coffee, Tea, or Free Drink
*Fat Choice

ANYTIME SNACK
2 Bread Choices
1 Cup Skim Milk
*Fat Choice

LUNCH
Free Salad
1 Vegetable Choice
1/2 Cup Beans or 1 Bread Choice
1 Fruit Choice
Coffee, Tea, or Free Drink
*Fat Choice

DINNER
1 Main Dish Choice
1 Side Dish Choice
1 Vegetable Choice
Free Salad
Coffee, Tea, or Free Drink
*Fat Choice

*** Fat choices are
optional and
should TOTAL no
more than 15 grams
of fat per day.**

P.M. SNACK
1 Fruit Choice or
4 Ounces Dry or Semi-dry Wine or
2 Cups Air-popped Popcorn

Today's Food Could Be	*Today's Fat Grams*

BREAKFAST

1 cup puffed wheat

1½ cups strawberries

1 cup skim milk

coffee

*_____

ANYTIME SNACK

1 cup skim milk

cinnamon toast: 2 slices wheat toast

*   2 tsp regular margarine   8

      1 tsp cinnamon/sugar mix

LUNCH

Free Salad

1 cup raw carrot sticks

1 slice rye bread

⅙ crenshaw melon

seltzer

* 2 oz lean roast beef   4

DINNER

6 oz grilled halibut steak

3/4 cup steamed buckwheat groats

1 cup steamed peas

Free Salad

coffee

* cooking spray   2

P.M. SNACK

4 oz wine

                          Today's Fat Choices Total   14

Getting Ahead
MENU SAMPLE—DAY 14

Menu Pattern

BREAKFAST
1 Ounce Cereal Choice
1 Fruit Choice
1 Cup Skim Milk
Coffee, Tea, or Free Drink
***Fat Choice**

ANYTIME SNACK
2 Bread Choices
1 Cup Skim Milk
***Fat Choice**

LUNCH
Free Salad
1 Vegetable Choice
1/2 Cup Beans or 1 Bread Choice
1 Fruit Choice
Coffee, Tea, or Free Drink
***Fat Choice**

DINNER
1 Main Dish Choice
1 Side Dish Choice
1 Vegetable Choice
Free Salad
Coffee, Tea, or Free Drink
***Fat Choice**

* Fat choices are optional and should TOTAL no more than 15 grams of fat per day.

P.M. SNACK
1 Fruit Choice or
4 Ounces Dry or Semi-dry Wine or
2 Cups Air-popped Popcorn

*Today's Food
Could Be*

BREAKFAST

1 oz oat bran

4 prunes

1 cup skim milk

coffee

*_____   _____

ANYTIME SNACK

1 plain bagel

1 cup skim milk

*_____   _____

LUNCH

Free Salad

1 cup steamed green beans

1/2 cup cooked white beans

1 small banana

iced tea

* 1 tbsp olive oil   14

DINNER

3 oz roasted pork tenderloin

1 large baked potato

1 cup steamed yellow squash

Free Salad

tea

*_____   _____

P.M. SNACK

1/2 cup fruit cocktail

Today's Fat Choices Total   14

Getting Ahead
MENU WORKSHEET—DAY 15

Menu Pattern

BREAKFAST
1 Ounce Cereal Choice
1 Fruit Choice
1 Cup Skim Milk
Coffee, Tea, or Free Drink
***Fat Choice**

ANYTIME SNACK
2 Bread Choices
1 Cup Skim Milk
***Fat Choice**

LUNCH
Free Salad
1 Vegetable Choice
1/2 Cup Beans or 1 Bread Choice
1 Fruit Choice
Coffee, Tea, or Free Drink
***Fat Choice**

DINNER
1 Main Dish Choice
1 Side Dish Choice
1 Vegetable Choice
Free Salad
Coffee, Tea, or Free Drink
***Fat Choice**

* Fat choices are optional and should TOTAL no more than 15 grams of fat per day.

P.M. SNACK
1 Fruit Choice or
4 Ounces Dry or Semi-dry Wine or
2 Cups Air-popped Popcorn

*Today's Food
Could Be*

BREAKFAST

_____

_____

_____

_____

*_____

ANYTIME SNACK

_____

_____

*_____

LUNCH

_____

_____

_____

_____

_____

*_____

DINNER

_____

_____

_____

_____

_____

*_____

P.M. SNACK

_____

*Today's
Fat Grams*

_____

_____

_____

_____

Today's Fat Choices Total   _____

Getting Ahead
MENU WORKSHEET—DAY 16

Menu Pattern

BREAKFAST
1 Ounce Cereal Choice
1 Fruit Choice
1 Cup Skim Milk
Coffee, Tea, or Free Drink
***Fat Choice**

ANYTIME SNACK
2 Bread Choices
1 Cup Skim Milk
***Fat Choice**

LUNCH
Free Salad
1 Vegetable Choice
1/2 Cup Beans or 1 Bread Choice
1 Fruit Choice
Coffee, Tea, or Free Drink
***Fat Choice**

DINNER
1 Main Dish Choice
1 Side Dish Choice
1 Vegetable Choice
Free Salad
Coffee, Tea, or Free Drink
***Fat Choice**

* Fat choices are optional and should TOTAL no more than 15 grams of fat per day.

P.M. SNACK
1 Fruit Choice or
4 Ounces Dry or Semi-dry Wine or
2 Cups Air-popped Popcorn

Today's Food
Could Be

Today's
Fat Grams

BREAKFAST

_____

_____

_____

_____

*_____   _____

ANYTIME SNACK

_____

_____

*_____   _____

LUNCH

_____

_____

_____

_____

_____

*_____   _____

DINNER

_____

_____

_____

_____

_____

*_____   _____

P.M. SNACK

_____

Today's Fat Choices Total   _____

Menu Pattern

BREAKFAST
1 Ounce Cereal Choice
1 Fruit Choice
1 Cup Skim Milk
Coffee, Tea, or Free Drink
*Fat Choice

ANYTIME SNACK
2 Bread Choices
1 Cup Skim Milk
*Fat Choice

LUNCH
Free Salad
1 Vegetable Choice
$1/2$ Cup Beans or 1 Bread Choice
1 Fruit Choice
Coffee, Tea, or Free Drink
*Fat Choice

DINNER
1 Main Dish Choice
1 Side Dish Choice
1 Vegetable Choice
Free Salad
Coffee, Tea, or Free Drink
*Fat Choice

* Fat choices are optional and should TOTAL no more than 15 grams of fat per day.

P.M. SNACK
1 Fruit Choice or
4 Ounces Dry or Semi-dry Wine or
2 Cups Air-popped Popcorn

*Today's Food
Could Be*

*Today's
Fat Grams*

BREAKFAST

_____

_____

_____

_____

*_____   _____

ANYTIME SNACK

_____

_____

*_____   _____

LUNCH

_____

_____

_____

_____

_____

*_____   _____

DINNER

_____

_____

_____

_____

_____

*_____   _____

P.M. SNACK

_____

Today's Fat Choices Total   _____

Getting Ahead
MENU WORKSHEET—DAY 18

Menu Pattern

BREAKFAST
1 Ounce Cereal Choice
1 Fruit Choice
1 Cup Skim Milk
Coffee, Tea, or Free Drink
***Fat Choice**

ANYTIME SNACK
2 Bread Choices
1 Cup Skim Milk
***Fat Choice**

LUNCH
Free Salad
1 Vegetable Choice
½ Cup Beans or 1 Bread Choice
1 Fruit Choice
Coffee, Tea, or Free Drink
***Fat Choice**

DINNER
1 Main Dish Choice
1 Side Dish Choice
1 Vegetable Choice
Free Salad
Coffee, Tea, or Free Drink
***Fat Choice**

P.M. SNACK
1 Fruit Choice or
4 Ounces Dry or Semi-dry Wine or
2 Cups Air-popped Popcorn

** Fat choices are
optional and
should TOTAL no
more than 15 grams
of fat per day.*

*Today's Food
Could Be*

*Today's
Fat Grams*

BREAKFAST

_____

_____

_____

_____

*_____   _____

ANYTIME SNACK

_____

_____

*_____   _____

LUNCH

_____

_____

_____

_____

_____

*_____   _____

DINNER

_____

_____

_____

_____

*_____   _____

P.M. SNACK

_____

_____

Today's Fat Choices Total   _____

Getting Ahead
MENU WORKSHEET—DAY 19

Menu Pattern

BREAKFAST
1 Ounce Cereal Choice
1 Fruit Choice
1 Cup Skim Milk
Coffee, Tea, or Free Drink
***Fat Choice**

ANYTIME SNACK
2 Bread Choices
1 Cup Skim Milk
***Fat Choice**

LUNCH
Free Salad
1 Vegetable Choice
1/2 Cup Beans or 1 Bread Choice
1 Fruit Choice
Coffee, Tea, or Free Drink
***Fat Choice**

DINNER
1 Main Dish Choice
1 Side Dish Choice
1 Vegetable Choice
Free Salad
Coffee, Tea, or Free Drink
***Fat Choice**

* *Fat choices are
optional and
should TOTAL no
more than 15 grams
of fat per day.*

P.M. SNACK
1 Fruit Choice or
4 Ounces Dry or Semi-dry Wine or
2 Cups Air-popped Popcorn

*Today's Food
Could Be*

*Today's
Fat Grams*

BREAKFAST

_____
_____
_____
_____
*_____   _____

ANYTIME SNACK

_____
_____
*_____   _____

LUNCH

_____
_____
_____
_____
_____
*_____   _____

DINNER

_____
_____
_____
_____
_____
*_____   _____

P.M. SNACK

_____

Today's Fat Choices Total   _____

Getting Ahead
MENU WORKSHEET—DAY 20

Menu Pattern

BREAKFAST
1 Ounce Cereal Choice
1 Fruit Choice
1 Cup Skim Milk
Coffee, Tea, or Free Drink
***Fat Choice**

ANYTIME SNACK
2 Bread Choices
1 Cup Skim Milk
***Fat Choice**

LUNCH
Free Salad
1 Vegetable Choice
¹/₂ Cup Beans or 1 Bread Choice
1 Fruit Choice
Coffee, Tea, or Free Drink
***Fat Choice**

DINNER
1 Main Dish Choice
1 Side Dish Choice
1 Vegetable Choice
Free Salad
Coffee, Tea, or Free Drink
***Fat Choice**

* *Fat choices are optional and should TOTAL no more than 15 grams of fat per day.*

P.M. SNACK
1 Fruit Choice or
4 Ounces Dry or Semi-dry Wine or
2 Cups Air-popped Popcorn

*Today's Food
Could Be*

*Today's
Fat Grams*

BREAKFAST

_____

_____

_____

_____

*_____   _____

ANYTIME SNACK

_____

_____

*_____   _____

LUNCH

_____

_____

_____

_____

_____

*_____   _____

DINNER

_____

_____

_____

_____

*_____   _____

P.M. SNACK

_____

Today's Fat Choices Total   _____

Getting Ahead
MENU WORKSHEET—DAY 21

Menu Pattern

BREAKFAST
1 Ounce Cereal Choice
1 Fruit Choice
1 Cup Skim Milk
Coffee, Tea, or Free Drink
***Fat Choice**

ANYTIME SNACK
2 Bread Choices
1 Cup Skim Milk
***Fat Choice**

LUNCH
Free Salad
1 Vegetable Choice
1/2 Cup Beans or 1 Bread Choice
1 Fruit Choice
Coffee, Tea, or Free Drink
***Fat Choice**

DINNER
1 Main Dish Choice
1 Side Dish Choice
1 Vegetable Choice
Free Salad
Coffee, Tea, or Free Drink
***Fat Choice**

* Fat choices are optional and should TOTAL no more than 15 grams of fat per day.

P.M. SNACK
1 Fruit Choice or
4 Ounces Dry or Semi-dry Wine or
2 Cups Air-popped Popcorn

*Today's Food
Could Be*

*Today's
Fat Grams*

BREAKFAST

_____
_____
_____
_____
* _____   _____

ANYTIME SNACK

_____
_____
* _____   _____

LUNCH

_____
_____
_____
_____
_____
* _____   _____

DINNER

_____
_____
_____
_____
_____
* _____   _____

P.M. SNACK

_____

Today's Fat Choices Total   _____

Menu Pattern

BREAKFAST

1 Ounce Cereal Choice

1 Fruit Choice

1 Cup Skim Milk

Coffee, Tea, or Free Drink

***Fat Choice**

ANYTIME SNACK

2 Bread Choices

1 Cup Skim Milk

***Fat Choice**

LUNCH

Free Salad

1 Vegetable Choice

½ Cup Beans or 1 Bread Choice

1 Fruit Choice

Coffee, Tea, or Free Drink

***Fat Choice**

DINNER

1 Main Dish Choice

1 Side Dish Choice

1 Vegetable Choice

Free Salad

Coffee, Tea, or Free Drink

***Fat Choice**

* Fat choices are optional and should TOTAL no more than 15 grams of fat per day.

P.M. SNACK

1 Fruit Choice or

4 Ounces Dry or Semi-dry Wine or

2 Cups Air-popped Popcorn

Today's Food
Could Be

BREAKFAST

_____
_____
_____
_____
*_____   _____

ANYTIME SNACK

_____
_____
*_____   _____

LUNCH

_____
_____
_____
_____
_____
*_____   _____

DINNER

_____
_____
_____
_____
*_____   _____

P.M. SNACK

_____

Today's Fat Choices Total   _____

Getting Ahead
MENU WORKSHEET—DAY 23

Menu Pattern

BREAKFAST
1 Ounce Cereal Choice
1 Fruit Choice
1 Cup Skim Milk
Coffee, Tea, or Free Drink
***Fat Choice**

ANYTIME SNACK
2 Bread Choices
1 Cup Skim Milk
***Fat Choice**

LUNCH
Free Salad
1 Vegetable Choice
½ Cup Beans or 1 Bread Choice
1 Fruit Choice
Coffee, Tea, or Free Drink
***Fat Choice**

DINNER
1 Main Dish Choice
1 Side Dish Choice
1 Vegetable Choice
Free Salad
Coffee, Tea, or Free Drink
***Fat Choice**

*** *Fat choices are
optional and
should TOTAL no
more than 15 grams
of fat per day.***

P.M. SNACK
1 Fruit Choice or
4 Ounces Dry or Semi-dry Wine or
2 Cups Air-popped Popcorn

*Today's Food
Could Be*

*Today's
Fat Grams*

BREAKFAST

_____
_____
_____
_____
*_____   _____

ANYTIME SNACK

_____
_____
*_____   _____

LUNCH

_____
_____
_____
_____
_____
*_____   _____

DINNER

_____
_____
_____
_____
*_____   _____

P.M. SNACK

_____

Today's Fat Choices Total   _____

Getting Ahead
MENU WORKSHEET—DAY 24

Menu Pattern

BREAKFAST
1 Ounce Cereal Choice
1 Fruit Choice
1 Cup Skim Milk
Coffee, Tea, or Free Drink
***Fat Choice**

ANYTIME SNACK
2 Bread Choices
1 Cup Skim Milk
***Fat Choice**

LUNCH
Free Salad
1 Vegetable Choice
1/2 Cup Beans or 1 Bread Choice
1 Fruit Choice
Coffee, Tea, or Free Drink
***Fat Choice**

DINNER
1 Main Dish Choice
1 Side Dish Choice
1 Vegetable Choice
Free Salad
Coffee, Tea, or Free Drink
***Fat Choice**

P.M. SNACK
1 Fruit Choice or
4 Ounces Dry or Semi-dry Wine or
2 Cups Air-popped Popcorn

** Fat choices are
optional and
should TOTAL no
more than 15 grams
of fat per day.*

210 · *Getting Ahead*

Today's Food
Could Be

Today's
Fat Grams

BREAKFAST

_____

_____

_____

_____

*_____   _____

ANYTIME SNACK

_____

_____

*_____   _____

LUNCH

_____

_____

_____

_____

_____

_____

*_____   _____

DINNER

_____

_____

_____

_____

*_____   _____

P.M. SNACK

_____

Today's Fat Choices Total   _____

Getting Ahead
MENU WORKSHEET—DAY 25

Menu Pattern

BREAKFAST
1 Ounce Cereal Choice
1 Fruit Choice
1 Cup Skim Milk
Coffee, Tea, or Free Drink
***Fat Choice**

ANYTIME SNACK
2 Bread Choices
1 Cup Skim Milk
***Fat Choice**

LUNCH
Free Salad
1 Vegetable Choice
½ Cup Beans or 1 Bread Choice
1 Fruit Choice
Coffee, Tea, or Free Drink
***Fat Choice**

DINNER
1 Main Dish Choice
1 Side Dish Choice
1 Vegetable Choice
Free Salad
Coffee, Tea, or Free Drink
***Fat Choice**

*** Fat choices are
optional and
should TOTAL no
more than 15 grams
of fat per day.*

P.M. SNACK
1 Fruit Choice or
4 Ounces Dry or Semi-dry Wine or
2 Cups Air-popped Popcorn

Today's Food
Could Be

Today's
Fat Grams

BREAKFAST

_____

_____

_____

_____

*_____   _____

ANYTIME SNACK

_____

_____

*_____   _____

LUNCH

_____

_____

_____

_____

_____

*_____   _____

DINNER

_____

_____

_____

_____

_____

*_____   _____

P.M. SNACK

_____

Today's Fat Choices Total   _____

Menu Pattern

BREAKFAST
1 Ounce Cereal Choice
1 Fruit Choice
1 Cup Skim Milk
Coffee, Tea, or Free Drink
***Fat Choice**

ANYTIME SNACK
2 Bread Choices
1 Cup Skim Milk
***Fat Choice**

LUNCH
Free Salad
1 Vegetable Choice
1/2 Cup Beans or 1 Bread Choice
1 Fruit Choice
Coffee, Tea, or Free Drink
***Fat Choice**

DINNER
1 Main Dish Choice
1 Side Dish Choice
1 Vegetable Choice
Free Salad
Coffee, Tea, or Free Drink
***Fat Choice**

*** *Fat choices are
optional and
should TOTAL no
more than 15 grams
of fat per day.***

P.M. SNACK
1 Fruit Choice or
4 Ounces Dry or Semi-dry Wine or
2 Cups Air-popped Popcorn

*Today's Food
Could Be*

*Today's
Fat Grams*

BREAKFAST

_____
_____
_____
_____
*_____   _____

ANYTIME SNACK

_____
_____
*_____   _____

LUNCH

_____
_____
_____
_____
_____
*_____   _____

DINNER

_____
_____
_____
_____
_____
*_____   _____

P.M. SNACK

_____
              Today's Fat Choices Total   _____

Getting Ahead
MENU WORKSHEET—DAY 27

Menu Pattern

BREAKFAST
1 Ounce Cereal Choice
1 Fruit Choice
1 Cup Skim Milk
Coffee, Tea, or Free Drink
***Fat Choice**

ANYTIME SNACK
2 Bread Choices
1 Cup Skim Milk
***Fat Choice**

LUNCH
Free Salad
1 Vegetable Choice
½ Cup Beans or 1 Bread Choice
1 Fruit Choice
Coffee, Tea, or Free Drink
***Fat Choice**

DINNER
1 Main Dish Choice
1 Side Dish Choice
1 Vegetable Choice
Free Salad
Coffee, Tea, or Free Drink
***Fat Choice**

P.M. SNACK
1 Fruit Choice or
4 Ounces Dry or Semi-dry Wine or
2 Cups Air-popped Popcorn

* *Fat choices are optional and should TOTAL no more than 15 grams of fat per day.*

*Today's Food
Could Be*

*Today's
Fat Grams*

BREAKFAST

_____

_____

_____

_____

*_____   _____

ANYTIME SNACK

_____

_____

*_____   _____

LUNCH

_____

_____

_____

_____

_____

*_____   _____

DINNER

_____

_____

_____

_____

*_____   _____

P.M. SNACK

_____

Today's Fat Choices Total   _____

Getting Ahead
MENU WORKSHEET—DAY 28

Menu Pattern

BREAKFAST
1 Ounce Cereal Choice
1 Fruit Choice
1 Cup Skim Milk
Coffee, Tea, or Free Drink
***Fat Choice**

ANYTIME SNACK
2 Bread Choices
1 Cup Skim Milk
***Fat Choice**

LUNCH
Free Salad
1 Vegetable Choice
½ Cup Beans or 1 Bread Choice
1 Fruit Choice
Coffee, Tea, or Free Drink
***Fat Choice**

DINNER
1 Main Dish Choice
1 Side Dish Choice
1 Vegetable Choice
Free Salad
Coffee, Tea, or Free Drink
***Fat Choice**

* Fat choices are optional and should TOTAL no more than 15 grams of fat per day.

P.M. SNACK
1 Fruit Choice or
4 Ounces Dry or Semi-dry Wine or
2 Cups Air-popped Popcorn

218 · *Getting Ahead*

Today's Food
Could Be

Today's
Fat Grams

BREAKFAST

_____

_____

_____

_____

* _____   _____

ANYTIME SNACK

_____

_____

* _____   _____

LUNCH

_____

_____

_____

_____

_____

* _____   _____

DINNER

_____

_____

_____

_____

_____

* _____   _____

P.M. SNACK

_____

                    Today's Fat Choices Total   _____

Getting Ahead
FOOD LISTS

These lists make it easier for you to attack your fat. Refer to them whenever your Getting Ahead menu indicates that you have a food choice to make.

During Getting Ahead, use:

Getting Ahead Fat Choices · Side Dish Choices
Cereal Choices   Free Salad Fixings
Fruit Choices   Free Drinks
Bread Choices   Getting Ahead Free Sweets
Vegetable Choices   Free Condiments
Main Dish Choices

Getting Ahead FAT CHOICES

Food	*Portion*	*Grams of Fat*
Almonds	12 nuts (½ ounce)	8
American cheese	1 ounce	9
Avocado	¼ avocado	7
Bacon, cooked	1 slice	3
Blue cheese	1 ounce	9
Brie cheese	1 ounce	8
Butter	1 tablespoon	12
Butter	1 teaspoon	4
Butter, whipped	1 ounce	15
Butter, whipped	1 tablespoon	9
Butter, whipped	1 teaspoon	3
Camembert cheese	1 ounce	6
Cheddar cheese	1 ounce	9
Colby cheese	1 ounce	9
Cooking spray	2.5-second spray	1
Corn oil	1 tablespoon	14
Corn oil	1 teaspoon	5
Cottage cheese, 1% fat	½ cup	1
Cottage cheese, 2% fat	½ cup	4
Cottage cheese, creamed	½ cup	5
Cream (half-and-half)	2 tablespoons	4
Cream cheese, light, reduced fat	1 ounce	5
Cream cheese, regular	1 ounce	10
Cream cheese, whipped	1 ounce	10
Edam cheese	1 ounce	8
Egg	1	6
Farmer cheese	1 ounce	8
Feta cheese	1 ounce	6
Gouda cheese	1 ounce	8
Half-and-half (cream)	2 tablespoons	4
Ham, lean	1 ounce	1
Ham, regular	1 ounce	3
Margarine	1 tablespoon	12
Margarine	1 teaspoon	4
Margarine, diet	1 tablespoon	6
Margarine, diet	1 teaspoon	2

Margarine, soft	1 tablespoon	11
Margarine, whipped	1 tablespoon	7
Mayonnaise	1 tablespoon	11
Mayonnaise	1 teaspoon	4
Mayonnaise, reduced calorie	1 tablespoon	5
Mayonnaise, reduced calorie	1 teaspoon	2
Mozzarella cheese	1 ounce	6
Mozzarella cheese, part skim	1 ounce	5
Muenster cheese	1 ounce	9
Neufchâtel cheese	1 ounce	7
Olive oil	1 tablespoon	14
Olive oil	1 teaspoon	5
Olives, black	2 large	4
Parmesan cheese, grated	1 tablespoon	2
Peanut butter, chunky	1 tablespoon	8
Peanut butter, smooth	1 tablespoon	8
Peanuts	20 nuts (½ ounce)	7
Provolone cheese	1 ounce	8
Ricotta cheese, part skim	¼ cup	5
Ricotta cheese, whole milk	¼ cup	8
Roast beef, lean	1 ounce	2
Salad dressing, blue cheese	1 tablespoon	8
Salad dressing, French	1 tablespoon	6
Salad dressing, French, reduced calorie	1 tablespoon	1
Salad dressing, Italian	1 tablespoon	7
Salad dressing, Italian, reduced calorie	1 tablespoon	2
Sour cream	¼ cup	12
Sour cream	1 tablespoon	3
Sour cream, imitation	1 tablespoon	3
Swiss cheese	1 ounce	8
Tuna, canned in water	2 ounces	1
Turkey, light meat	1 ounce	1
Walnuts	8 halves (½ ounce)	8
Yogurt, low-fat, any flavor	6–8 ounces	2

Getting Ahead CEREAL CHOICES

For Getting Ahead, choose one of these, or any cereal that contains two grams of fat or less in each one-ounce serving.

100% Bran with Oat Bran NABISCO
100% Oat Bran SKINNERS
7-Grain Crunchy LOMA LINDA
7-Grain No Sugar Added LOMA LINDA
Cheerios GENERAL MILLS
Cheerios, Apple Cinnamon GENERAL MILLS
Cheerios, Honey Nut GENERAL MILLS
Common Sense Oat Bran KELLOGG'S
Cracklin' Oat Bran KELLOGG'S
Fortified Oat Flakes POST
Honey Bunches of Oats POST
Hot Bran Hot Cereal HEALTH VALLEY
Instant Oatmeal QUAKER
Instant Oatmeal Regular EREWHON
Instant Oatmeal Regular RALSTON
Instant Oatmeal with Apples & Cinnamon QUAKER
Instant Oatmeal with Cinnamon & Spice RALSTON
Instant Oatmeal with Cinnamon & Spices QUAKER
Instant Oatmeal with Maple & Brown Sugar QUAKER
Instant Oatmeal with Maple & Brown Sugar RALSTON
Irish Oatmeal, Quick Cooking McCANN'S
Kashi, 5 Bran Instant Cereal KASHI
Kashi, Lightly Puffed KASHI
Kashi, The Breakfast Pilaf KASHI
Nutrific Oatmeal Flakes KELLOGG'S
Oat Bran MOTHER'S
Oat Bran QUAKER
Oat Bran Crunch KOLLIN
Oat Bran Flakes HEALTH VALLEY
Oat Bran Options RALSTON
Oat Bran O's HEALTH VALLEY
Oat Bran O's Fruit & Nuts HEALTH VALLEY
Oat Bran with Toasted Wheat Germ EREWHON
Oat Meal McCANN'S
Oat Squares QUAKER

Oatmeal Maple Flavor MAYPO
Oatmeal Raisin Crisp GENERAL MILLS
Oatmeal Swirlers GENERAL MILLS
Old Fashioned Oatmeal QUAKER
Puffed Kashi KASHI
Quaker Extra Apples & Spice QUAKER
Quaker Extra Raisins & Cinnamon QUAKER
Quaker Extra Regular QUAKER
Quick Oatmeal RALSTON
Quick Oats ROMAN MEAL
Regular Oatmeal RALSTON
Total Instant Oatmeal Regular GENERAL MILLS
Total Oatmeal Quick GENERAL MILLS
Wholesome 'n Hearty Instant Oat Bran Hot Cereal NABISCO
Wholesome 'n Hearty Instant Oat Bran Hot Cereal, Honey NABISCO
Wholesome 'n Hearty Instant Oat Bran Hot Cereal, Apple Cinnamon
    NABISCO
Wholesome 'n Hearty Oat Bran Hot Cereal NABISCO

Getting Ahead FRUIT CHOICES

Use fresh fruits or canned fruits unless otherwise noted. (Portion sizes recommended are to help you learn the "Thin Habit" of eating moderate servings.)

Fruit	*Serving Size*
Apple	1 medium
Apricots	4 small, fresh **or** 8 halves, dried
Asian pear	1 medium
Banana	1 small **or** ½ medium
Blackberries	1 cup
Blueberries	1 cup
Cantaloupe	½ small **or** ¼ medium **or** 1 cup, cubed
Carambola	2 fruits
Casaba	1½ cups
Cherimoya	⅙ fruit
Cherries	15 fruits
Clementine	2 fruits
Cranberries, raw	¾ cup
Crenshaw	⅙ fruit

Getting Ahead FRUIT CHOICES (*cont.*)

Fruit	Serving Size
Fig	2 small or 1 medium
Fruit cocktail	½ cup
Gooseberries	1 cup
Grapefruit	1 medium
Grapes	20 (1 small bunch)
Guava	1 fruit
Honeydew	⅛ melon or 1 cup, cubed
Kiwi	1 fruit
Lychee	10 fruits
Loquat	10 fruits
Mandarin orange sections	½ cup
Mango	½ fruit
Nectarine	1 large or 2 small
Orange	1 large
Papaya	½ fruit
Peach	1 large or 2 small
Pear	1 medium
Persian melon	¼ medium or 1 cup, cubed
Persimmon	1 large
Pineapple	1 cup fresh or ½ cup, canned
Plantain	⅓ cup
Plum	2 medium
Pomegranate	½ fruit
Pomelo	1 medium
Prunes	4 fruits
Raisins	2 tablespoons (⅛ cup)
Raspberries	1 cup
Rhubarb	¾ cup
Santa Claus melon	1/12 fruit
Sapodilla	½ fruit
Strawberries	1½ cups
Tamarind	10 fruits
Tangelo	1 fruit
Tangerine	2 fruits
Ugli fruit	1 medium
Watermelon	1 cup

Getting Ahead BREAD CHOICES

Each of the following equals 1 Bread Choice. (Portion sizes recommended are to help you learn the "Thin Habit" of eating moderate servings.)

Bagel, any variety	½ bagel*
Breadsticks, plain	2 breadsticks
Brown bread, canned	½ slice*
Brown bread with raisins, canned	½ slice*
Cinnamon bread	½ slice*
Cracklebread	4 pieces
English muffin	½ muffin*
French bread	1 slice (1-inch thick)
Hamburger roll	½ roll*
Hard roll	½ roll*
Hot dog bun	½ bun*
Italian bread	1 slice (1-inch thick)
Melba toast, any variety	2 pieces
Norwegian crispbread	3 pieces
Pita bread	1 pocket (6-inch diameter)
Pita, whole wheat	1 pocket (6-inch diameter)
Popcorn, air popped, unbuttered	2 cups
Pumpernickel	1 slice
Pumpernickel, snack loaf	4 slices
Raisin bread	½ slice*
Rice cakes, any variety	2 pieces
Rye, dill	1 slice
Rye, seeded	1 slice
Rye, snack loaf	4 slices
Rye, unseeded	1 slice
Wasa crispbread, any variety	2 pieces
Wheat bread	1 slice
White bread	1 slice
Whole-wheat bread	1 slice

*For these choices, 1 bagel, 1 roll, or 1 English muffin equals 2 Bread Choices.

Getting Ahead VEGETABLE CHOICES

The serving size for each Vegetable Choice is 1 cup. (Portion size rec-ommended is to help you learn the "Thin Habit" of eating moderate servings.)

Artichoke	Jerusalem artichoke	Squash, butternut
Asparagus	Jicama	Squash, cozelle
Bamboo shoots	Kale	Squash, crookneck
Beet greens	Leeks	Squash, cymling
Beets	Lima beans	Squash, delicious
Broccoli	Mixed vegetables	Squash, Hubbard
Brussels sprouts	Napa	Squash, pattypan
Butter beans	Okra	Squash, spaghetti
Carrot	Parsnips	Squash, straight-neck
Cauliflower	Pea pods	Squash, turban
Celery	Peas	Squash, yellow
Chayote	Pumpkin	Sugar snap peas
Collard greens	Rutabaga	Tomatillo
Corn	Salsify	Turnip
Daikon	Sauerkraut	Turnip greens
Dandelion greens	Snow peas	Water chestnuts
Eggplant	Squash, acorn	Wax beans
Green beans	Squash, banana	Yucca
Italian green beans	Squash, buttercup	Zucchini

Getting Ahead MAIN DISH CHOICES

Different portion sizes are given for Main Dish Choices because the foods on this list vary in fat content.

Choice	Serving Size After Cooking
Beef, brisket, lean only	3 ounces
Beef, eye round	3 ounces
Beef, round	3 ounces
Beef, round, ground	3 ounces
Beef, sirloin	3 ounces
Beef, tenderloin (fillet)	3 ounces
Canadian bacon	4 ounces

Catfish, fillet	4 ounces
Chicken breast, no skin	½ breast
Chicken leg and thigh, no skin	1
Chicken, white meat, boneless	4 ounces
Chipped beef	3 ounces
Clams, canned in water	5 ounces
Clams, fresh, shelled	5 ounces
Cod, fillet or steak	6 ounces
Cottage cheese, creamed	¾ cup
Cottage cheese, low-fat	1 cup
Crab, canned in water	4 ounces
Crab, fresh	4 ounces
Flank steak	3 ounces
Flounder, fillet	6 ounces
Grouper	6 ounces
Haddock, fillet	6 ounces
Halibut, fillet or steak	6 ounces
Ham, canned	4 ounces
Ham, cured	4 ounces
Ham, fresh	3 ounces
Herring, jarred in vinegar	3 ounces
Herring, smoked	3 ounces
Hot dog, chicken	1
Hot dog, turkey	1
Leg of lamb, boneless	3 ounces
Lobster, canned in water	6 ounces
Lobster, fresh	6 ounces
Mussels	4 ounces
Oysters, fresh	12–15
Perch, fillet	4 ounces
Pike, fillet	5 ounces
Pollack, fillet	6 ounces
Pork tenderloin	4 ounces
Pot cheese	¾ cup
Ricotta cheese, light	3 ounces
Ricotta cheese, part skim	3 ounces
Rockfish, fillet	5 ounces
Roughy, fillet	3 ounces
Salmon, canned	3 ounces
Salmon, fresh, fillet or steak	3 ounces

Getting Ahead MAIN DISH CHOICES (*cont.*)

Choice	Serving Size After Cooking
Salmon, smoked	3 ounces
Sardines, canned in mustard	6 medium
Sardines, canned in tomato sauce	6 medium
Sardines, canned in water	6 medium
Scallops, canned in water	4 ounces
Scallops, fresh	4 ounces
Scrod, fillet	6 ounces
Shellfish substitute (surimi)	4 ounces
Shrimp, canned in water	5 ounces
Shrimp, fresh	5 ounces
Snapper, fillet	6 ounces
Sole, fillet	6 ounces
Sturgeon, fresh, fillet or steak	4 ounces
Sturgeon, smoked	4 ounces
Swordfish, fillet or steak	4 ounces
Tilefish, fresh, fillet	5 ounces
Tuna, canned in water	1 individual can
Tuna, fresh, fillet or steak	4 ounces
Turkey, boneless, no skin	4 ounces
Turkey, lean, ground	3 ounces
Veal, chop, meat only	3 ounces
Veal, cutlet	3 ounces
Veal, ground	4 ounces
Whitefish, smoked	4 ounces

Getting Ahead SIDE DISH CHOICES

(Portion sizes recommended are to help you learn the "Thin Habit" of eating moderate servings.)

Choice	Serving Size
Adzuki beans, cooked	½ cup
Barley, cooked	¾ cup
Black-eyed peas, cooked	½ cup

Buckwheat groats, cooked	¾ cup
Bulgur, cooked	¾ cup
Chick-peas, cooked	½ cup
Couscous, cooked	¾ cup
Cowpeas, cooked	½ cup
Cracked wheat, cooked	¾ cup
Cranberry beans, cooked	½ cup
Great northern beans, cooked	½ cup
Hyacinth beans, cooked	½ cup
Kidney beans, cooked	½ cup
Lentils, cooked	½ cup
Lima beans, cooked	½ cup
Mixed-bean salad, jarred	¾ cup
Mung beans, cooked	½ cup
Navy beans, cooked	½ cup
Noodles, no-yolk or no-egg variety, cooked	¾ cup
Pasta, any shape, cooked	¾ cup
Pasta, carrot, any shape, cooked	¾ cup
Pasta, Jerusalem artichoke, any shape, cooked	¾ cup
Pasta, oat bran, any shape, cooked	¾ cup
Pasta, spinach, any shape, cooked	¾ cup
Pasta, tomato, any shape, cooked	¾ cup
Pasta, tricolor, any shape, cooked	¾ cup
Pasta, whole wheat, any shape, cooked	¾ cup
Pink beans, cooked	½ cup
Pinto beans, cooked	½ cup
Potato, baked	1 large
Potato, boiled	1 cup
Potatoes, mashed, no added fat	¾ cup
Rice, brown, cooked	¾ cup
Rice, white, cooked	¾ cup
Split peas, cooked	½ cup
Spaghetti, any shape, cooked	¾ cup
Spaghetti, whole wheat, any shape, cooked	¾ cup
Sweet potato, baked	1 medium
Sweet potato, boiled	¾ cup
Sweet potatoes, mashed, no added fat	½ cup
Wheat berries, cooked	¾ cup
White beans, cooked	½ cup

Getting Ahead SIDE DISH CHOICES (*cont.*)

Choice	Serving Size
Wild rice, cooked	¾ cup
Yam, baked	1 medium
Yams, mashed, no added fat	½ cup

Getting Ahead FREE SALAD FIXINGS

Alfalfa sprouts
Arugula
Basil, fresh
Bean sprouts
Bibb lettuce
Bok choy
Boston lettuce
Butterhead lettuce
Cabbage
Cabbage, Chinese
Cabbage, red
Cabbage, savoy
Celery
Chard
Chicory
Chives
Cilantro
Cress

Cucumber
Dill, fresh
Endive
Escarole
Fennel
Garden cress
Garlic
Green onions (scallions)
Hot peppers
Iceberg lettuce
Kale
Kohlrabi
Looseleaf lettuce
Mint, fresh
Mung bean sprouts
Mushrooms
Mustard greens
Onions, red

Onions, Spanish
Onions, Vidalia
Onions, white
Parsley, fresh
Peppers, green
Peppers, red
Peppers, yellow
Pimiento
Radicchio
Radishes
Red-leaf lettuce
Rocket
Romaine lettuce
Sorrel
Shallot
Spinach
Tomato
Watercress

Getting Ahead FREE DRINKS

Club soda
Diet soda
Drink mixes, sugar-free
Herbal tea
Instant onion soup, dry mix
Mineral water

Pero (coffee substitute)
Postum (coffee substitute)
Seltzer
Seltzer, flavored
Water

Getting Ahead FREE SWEETS

Apple butter
Brown sugar
Diet jam
Diet jelly
Fruit butter
Fruit-only preserves

Honey
Molasses
Powdered sugar
Prune butter
Raw sugar
Regular jam

Regular jelly
Sugar
Sugar-free gelatin
Sugar-free gum
Sugar-free hard candy
Sugar substitutes

Getting Ahead FREE CONDIMENTS

Use the following condiments to flavor, garnish, or prepare foods.

Beef broth, cubes or powdered
Butter-flavored sprinkles
Chicken broth, cubes or powdered
Chives
Garlic
Ginger root
Gremolata (see page 118)
Herbs, dried (see pages 67–69)
Herbs, fresh (see pages 67–69)
Horseradish
Hot sauce
Ketchup
Lemon
Lemon juice
Lime
Lime juice
Mustard, coarse grain
Mustard, Dijon
Mustard, lemon
Mustard, regular
Mustard, tarragon
No-oil salad dressing
Pepper
Picante sauce
Pickles, dill

Salsa
Salt-free seasoning mixes
Seasoned pepper
Shallot
Soy sauce, regular
Soy sauce, light
Spices (see pages 67–69)
Tabasco sauce
Tamari
Tomato paste
Teriyaki sauce
Vegetable broth, cubes or powdered
Vinegar
Vinegar, balsamic
Vinegar, cider
Vinegar, herb flavored
Vinegar, raspberry
Vinegar, rice
Vinegar, tarragon
Vinegar, wine
Watermelon rind pickles
Worcestershire sauce
Zero Dressing (see page 78)

9 *In Control*
FAT ATTACK PLAN PHASE THREE

We recently spoke with a client—a man we'll call Jim—who had originally come to us simply because he had wanted to lose weight. "Fifty pounds," he'd said. "Let's just get it off." Dark-eyed and handsome in spite of his heft, he'd been motivated partly by vanity, and a lot by his wife. Although it probably hadn't been easy for him, he'd finally decided to do something about his expanding waistline.

We structured a workable diet for Jim—and even built in a beer for him to have each day after he left his job. That little break was important to him, and it was equally important to us to give him a plan he could enjoy.

Jim succeeded admirably. He reached his goal in less than eight months, and during that time we often heard how happy his wife was to be giving away the clothes that he had "ungrown."

Naturally, the eating plan we put Jim on was a low-fat one. We wanted to help him lose weight and this was the best way to do it. Fortunately for Jim he was basically in good health, and we wanted to be sure he stayed that way. The interesting part was that, at the time, he didn't care about the other benefits of his low-fat eating plan. He met our tried-and-true advice about the good-health virtues of attacking his fat with patient smiles but little interest. Whatever we were doing for him was just fine with him, as long as it made him look better, and by the time he'd reached his target weight he was a very happy man.

A few more months passed and we received a call from Jim, who reported that he'd kept the weight off by carefully watching the amount of fat in his diet. But he had even better news. He'd just gotten the results of his annual company physical. Not only was the doctor thrilled to see that Jim's weight had gone down considerably, but Jim himself was delighted to see what else had gone down since his last examination: His blood pressure, his cholesterol, and his triglycerides had all taken a significant nose dive. He was like a kid with a good report card.

"Now will you listen to us?" we asked, laughing. "We *told* you it works."

"It sure does," Jim replied. "I feel terrific!"

As well he should, because Jim could finally see that *all* the pieces were now in place—and that he'd put them there. Best of all, he was obviously succeeding in keeping them there. Yes, he'd learned how to control his weight, but he'd never realized, until he took his physical, exactly how *much* control he really had.

What It's All About

The control *is* in your hands! You can maintain your weight, and reduce your risk for serious illnesses, such as cancer, hypertension, heart disease, and diabetes, just by being "In Control." If you've already been through one or even two phases of the Fat Attack Plan, you've seen what it can do for you because *you* made it work. Like Jim, you've come a long way and you're ready now to enjoy the benefits of your hard work.

Even if you're starting out with In Control, your objectives are the same. You know your weight is good, and you know what your health risks are. Your job now is to make things better and to keep them that way.

Right now you're committed to good health—but will you still be a month from now, or a year from now? When you set up a lifelong eating plan it has to do more than ensure your good health. It has to be fun and flexible, and it has to work in *your* life, as Jim's did in his. If how you eat can't do that, you won't be eating that way for long—no matter how healthy it is.

That lack of flexibility is one of the reasons why so many diets fail and why so many dieters—even if they've lost weight—end up right back at Square One. But the Fat Attack Plan isn't like "so many diets." For one thing, it's not a "diet." Even if you haven't been through Super Start or Getting Ahead, you'll learn while In Control that the Fat Attack *Plan* is just that—an eating plan designed to teach you how to make sensible fat-food choices for weight control and lifelong good health.

Being In Control Is Different

The difference between In Control and the Super Start or Getting Ahead phases—the thing that *makes* it work in your life—is that now *you* make all the choices. You've already made the most important choice, the commitment to good health. Now that you've reached your target weight and you're ready to be In Control, you're going to see that maintaining your success is the easy part! When you're In Control, you continue to track the fat in the foods you eat, but now you do it in a much simpler way.

You won't be following Menu Patterns, the way you did on Super Start or Getting Ahead. The foods you eat will be entirely up to you. But you'll have the advantage—and the guidance—of working within the framework of a solid pattern for balanced eating, based on five groups of nutritious, good-tasting food—much of it fat free. And we'll provide you with a handy visual guide—we call it the "Fat Attack Target"—that you can refer to when making your food choices.

As you create your own daily menus from the five food groups, you'll also be tracking the fat in all the foods you eat, as you did in Getting Ahead. But now that you're In Control you're free to add as many as forty-five grams of fat to your menu each day if you're a woman, and sixty grams if you're a man. To help make tracking the fat in the foods you select as easy as possible, we've provided you with two special resources: a comprehensive list of Fat-Free Foods and an invaluable Fat Counter, which indicates the fat content in nearly one thousand popular foods.

The In Control Menu Planner

The In Control Menu Planner, which is based on five groups of healthy foods, is the best plan to follow each day to ensure good nutrition. If you've just finished Super Start or Getting Ahead, you've learned what a typical serving of any of these foods would be. If you're starting with In Control, refer to the Getting Ahead Food Lists on pages 222–33 for serving-size information.

- **Fruits and vegetables** (vitamin and mineral rich): Five servings a day recommended.

    The National Academy of Sciences recommends that we eat at least five servings of fruits and vegetables each day. While this may sound like a lot, it really isn't. Fat-free and loaded with fiber, fruits and vegetables—unadorned with fatty condiments—are *"free foods"* when you are In Control. That means you can eat as many servings as you want. Having one or two portions of fruits and/or vegetables at each meal, or having them as a snack, is a pleasant way to feel satisfied and get the nutrients you need.

    Citrus fruits, such as oranges, tangerines, and grapefruit, are especially rich sources of vitamin C. Papaya, tomatoes, red and green peppers, Brussels sprouts, broccoli, cantaloupe, strawberries, persimmons, and watermelon also have a lot of this vitamin. It's a good idea to eat one or two servings of these fruits each day because research suggests that vitamin C may bolster immune function.

Dark-green leafy vegetables and deep-yellow vegetables and fruits, such as broccoli, spinach, kale, collards, Romaine and red-leaf lettuce, carrots, sweet potatoes, mangoes, and apricots, are rich sources of beta-carotene, the plant form of vitamin A. And research shows that beta-carotene may be protective against many types of cancer, including lung cancer. It's smart to eat one or two servings of fruits and vegetables containing beta-carotene each day.

- **Bread, cereal, pasta, beans, rice, and other whole grains** (fiber rich): Three servings a day recommended. (See the sample menus on ideas about how to include these foods daily.)

  These foods are virtually fat free and particularly when eaten in their whole-grain form, contain an abundance of both soluble and insoluble fiber. Whole-grain varieties of bread, cereal, pasta, and brown rice are more filling and contain more vitamins, minerals, and fiber than those that are more processed, so choose whole grains whenever you can.

  Besides being satisfying and low in fat, beans are rich in soluble fiber, which has been shown to reduce levels of cholesterol and glucose (sugar) in the blood. Perhaps most valuable of all, eating high-fiber foods may prevent certain types of cancer, especially cancer of the colon.

- **Milk and yogurt** (calcium rich): Two servings a day recommended. (See the sample menus for ideas about how to include these foods daily.)

  Studies show that many women do not get enough calcium, and this can put them at increased risk for osteoporosis (adult bone loss). The two servings a day we suggest provide more than one-half of the recommended daily intake of this important mineral. Milk and yogurt are available in low-fat and fat-free varieties, making them easy to work into a healthy low-fat eating plan. The rest of your calcium can be provided by dark-green leafy vegetables, tofu, and—believe it or not—the bones in canned salmon and sardines.

- **Meat, fish, and poultry** (protein rich): Six ounces a day recommended. (See the sample menus for ideas about how to include these foods daily.)

  In their 1989 dietary guidelines for reducing the risk of chronic disease, the National Research Council recommends moderate protein intake for good health. Nevertheless, many Americans still eat more protein than they need. What they may not realize is that excess protein doesn't help the body because the kidneys have to work harder to process it.

Meat, fish, and poultry vary in the amount of fat they contain. Some fish—like cod—have very little fat, while others—like salmon—have much more. The same is true of meat; some cuts have more fat calories than protein calories. An average restaurant serving of fish or meat could be eight to ten ounces, which is more than you need. In addition to referring to Getting Ahead serving-size information on pages 228–30, you can easily estimate the size of a four-ounce portion. Just remember that a four-ounce piece of meat, fish, or poultry is about the same size as the palm of your hand, as long as it's about one-half inch thick—as thick as the place where your pinky joins your palm. For smaller portions, a deck of cards is equal in size to a piece weighing about three ounces.

IN CONTROL MENU PLANNER

Food Groups	Each Day Have
Vitamin-rich fruits and vegetables	5 servings
Fiber-rich bread, cereal, pasta, beans, rice, and other whole grains	3 servings
Calcium-rich milk and yogurt	2 servings
Protein-rich meat, fish, and poultry	6 ounces

Tracking Fat When You're In Control

Use the food groups above and the numbers of servings suggested as the basis for planning your meals when you're In Control. Herbs, spices, Free Condiments (see pages 67–69), Free Drinks (page 232), and Free Sweets (page 233) are yours to use whenever you wish in preparing your food or when serving it; they're "free" because they have no fat. You don't have to worry about them at all.

In fact, almost all the foods in the In Control Menu Planner are fat free or close to it, with the exception of "regular" dairy foods and some meats, fish, and poultry (many of the latter have hidden pockets of fat that can't be trimmed away). Obviously, if a food is fat free you can't—and don't need to—track the fat in it; but how do you track the fat in the protein foods you choose? And what about all the other fat foods you choose to include in your diet? How do you know how much of them you can eat without exceeding your daily fat allowance?

YOUR REFERENCE TOOLS

Experts recommend that Americans reduce the amount of fat they eat to 30 percent or less of their total calories. That's good advice, but following it can involve complicated math that most of us don't want to bother with on a daily basis. We offer an easy alternative: Simply keep track of the number of grams of fat in the foods you select each day with the help of the "Fat Counter" (which begins on page 300 and gives the fat content of many popular foods), and the Fat-Free Foods list (which begins on page 294 and lists the foods for which you *don't* have to track the fat).

If you're a woman, your daily fat intake shouldn't exceed forty-five grams; if you're a man, sixty grams is your allowance. When you keep your daily fat intake within these limits and follow the eating guidelines for In Control, your daily fat intake will automatically add up to less than 30 percent of all the calories you eat.

If you've finished Getting Ahead, you've already had some experience tracking fat—when you kept count of the fifteen grams of fat you added each day to your menu. Going into In Control, you'll probably need to formally keep track of your fat by writing it all down for only one or two weeks. After that, you'll find you've learned enough about fat in foods to be able to follow the 45/60-gram rule naturally and easily. You can still formally track your fat if you want, but if you'd prefer just to follow the general guidelines you can do that instead. If you need help in making the best food choices, you can consult the "Fat Attack Target."

We'll take a closer look at the Target in a moment, but for now just remember that until you're making your food decisions without having to think much about it, the Target is a handy visual guide that will help you immensely. One fast glance is all it takes to help you make a good decision.

If you're starting the Fat Attack Plan with In Control, be sure to carefully track the fat you eat for a full twenty-eight days. After you've done this, you can move along to using the Fat Attack Target as your only guide, counting fat grams once in a while, just to be sure you're staying In Control.

USING THE "FAT COUNTER"

Whether all this is new to you or not, just remember one thing: When *you're* In Control, *you* make all the choices. You can decide about everything you eat. Best of all, there are *no* foods that are "not allowed." You can enjoy all your favorites—in moderation, of course. Simply build your favorite food choices into your basic healthy Menu Planner and keep track of the fat they contain.

You'll probably find it easy to keep track of fat grams because, if you're like most Americans on most days, you probably eat the same foods over and over. Food consumption studies show that most of us eat only thirty-five different foods! Many of these foods, such as plain fruits, vegetables, cereal, rice, pasta, and beans, have virtually no fat. These are "free foods" (you don't have to track the fat in them), and you'll find them listed as Fat-Free Foods on pages 294–99. Naturally, the more of these foods you include in your diet the better.

But some fats are necessary in your diet, of course, and it's likely that most of the fat you eat comes from only a few choices—dairy foods, like milk and cheese; meat, fish, and poultry; butter, margarine, shortening, and other fats and oils, and foods that contain them. Many of these foods were on the Fat Choices list you became familiar with if you went through the Getting Ahead phase of the Fat Attack Plan. You'll find these and many other fat foods in the "Fat Counter," which starts on page 300.

The "Fat Counter" lists nearly one thousand foods and gives the grams of fat in a usual portion. All generic foods and many packaged ones are included. If you don't find the exact food you're looking for, choose another similar food. For example, if you can't find grated Romano cheese, use the figure for grated Parmesan cheese, a similar type.

The Fat Attack Target

If there's a way to condense the entire Fat Attack Plan into very little space, this is it! The "Fat Attack Target" says it all—at least, all of the most important things—and it can be your guide to making good food choices when you're In Control.

The concept of the Fat Attack Target is very simple. All foods at the center of the target are "free foods." *You can eat them whenever you wish and have as much of them as you want.* Fruits, vegetables, beans, bread, pasta, cereals, rice, and other grains can be eaten and enjoyed without giving their portion size or fat content a single thought. All these foods are rich in fiber, vitamins, and minerals, and they contain little or no fat.

The foods in the outer rings of the target are wholesome, too. You can certainly eat them. But they do contain fat, some more than others. How much of these foods you eat and how often you eat them have to be tracked. They're not free foods—there are limits to their use. When you're selecting foods from within the Fat Attack Target, pick foods that are closer to the center of the Target more often (they contain less fat) and foods in the outer rings less often (they contain more fat).

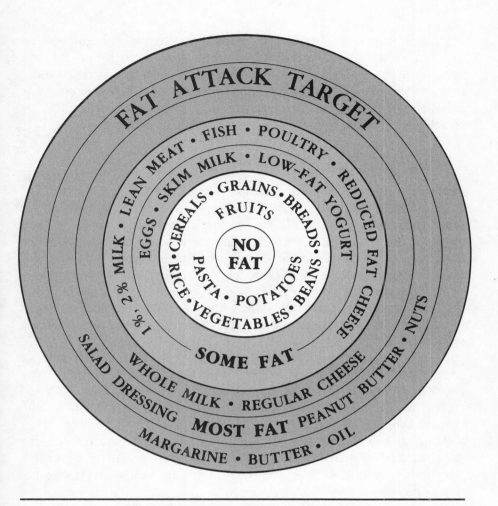

FAT ATTACK TARGET

- Foods near the center of the target—the bull's-eye—are "fat free." Fruits, vegetables, beans, rice, pasta, potatoes, breads, cereals, and grains are free foods. Have them as often as you wish. You do not need to track the fat in these foods.

- Foods in the middle rings contain "some fat." Skim milk, low-fat yogurt, 1% and 2% milk, reduced-fat cheese, eggs, and lean meat, fish, and poultry are good choices, too, but you need to track their fat. Use moderate amounts.

- Foods in the outermost rings, farthest from the bull's-eye, contain the "most fat." Use oil, butter, margarine, salad dressing, nuts, whole milk, and regular cheese less often.

You can use the Fat Attack Target anywhere. Use it as your guide when ordering in a fast-food restaurant or in an elegant French bistro. It will help you choose airline food or pick exotic cuisine at your destination. It doesn't matter if you don't know the name of a foreign cheese or unusual fruit. Using the Target tells you to eat as much of the fruit as you'd like but to eat only a modest amount of cheese.

Making Fat Choices

Let's take a careful look at all the choices in the Fat Attack Target.

The choices near the center of the target are low in fat; those in the outer rings are high in fat. This helps you separate high-fat foods from low-fat foods at a glance. You add more fat as you pick choices further from the center of the target. Therefore it makes good nutrition and health sense to make more choices from the center.

You'll notice that **skim milk** is close to the center of the target. It has the least amount of fat of any milk. So it's your best choice, with very little fat yet all the calcium and nutrients found in whole milk or other low-fat milks.

Low-fat yogurt is another good way to get calcium each day without adding much fat. Most brands carry a nutrition label, so you can quickly check to see which flavors are lowest in fat. Any low-fat variety is a good choice. Just be careful of those brands that use whole milk and cream; custard-style yogurts often do.

All **meat, fish, and poultry** contain some fat. Even well-trimmed, lean varieties have fat as part of the structure of the muscle. There are no "fat-free" varieties! Choosing lean cuts, trimming off visible fat, and eating moderate servings are the best ways to keep fat low.

Low-fat milks have varying amounts of fat: 1% or 2%. These have less fat than whole milk but more fat than skim milk (0%). If you drink a low-fat variety, that's fine—just keep track of the fat in it.

More and more companies are manufacturing **reduced-fat (or low-fat) cheeses**. Unfortunately, it's the fat in cheese that gives it its traditional creamy smoothness and melting qualities. Low-fat cheeses are often more rubbery in texture and don't melt and "run" as smoothly as regular cheese. Also, be careful of cheese substitutes; they're not low in fat. Although the butterfat has been removed, it's often replaced with oil, making the cheese substitute low in cholesterol but equally high in fat. Check the label: Whenever butterfat has been replaced with oil, the cheese must be labeled "imitation."

When you do pick low-fat cheeses, you should read the label carefully. If a claim like "low fat" or "low cholesterol" is made, the manufacturer is obligated to provide you with a complete nutrition label. Check to see how many grams of fat are in a one-ounce serving and compare it with the count in a traditional hard cheese, like cheddar. Then you can decide if you're really saving any fat by buying the "low-fat" version. The only real difference may be the cholesterol content.

A few cheeses are made in both low-fat and regular varieties. Mozzarella and part-skim mozzarella, ricotta and part-skim ricotta, cottage cheese and low-fat cottage cheese are a few. The part-skim or low-fat versions have less fat than the regular varieties. Other cheeses, like Jarlsberg (a skim-milk Swiss-type cheese) are not as low in fat as you're led to believe. If you buy Jarlsberg over regular Swiss, you save only one gram of fat per ounce. You can make similar comparisons with the help of the "Fat Counter," which begins on page 300.

You may be surprised to find out that **eggs** are not a high-fat food. One egg has five grams of fat, three of which are polyunsaturated, and two saturated. Eggs are often maligned because they contain too much cholesterol, but 1989 figures released by the U.S. Department of Agriculture show that the average egg contains almost 25 percent less cholesterol (213 milligrams) than once believed (274 milligrams). More accurate analysis techniques and newer feeding methods have both contributed to the lower figure.

Most nutrition experts, however, would still agree that it's not smart to eat an unlimited number of eggs, and this is why eggs are in the middle, "some fat" ring of your Fat Attack Target. They're a choice, but a choice that has limits; a sensible limit is three to four eggs a week.

A great "egg fact" that you should know is: All the fat and all the cholesterol in an egg is in the yolk. Egg white is fat free. If you'd like to have scrambled eggs one morning, instead of using two whole eggs, use one whole egg and the white of the second egg. Mix and scramble as you usually would, knowing that you just reduced the fat and the cholesterol by half. When you cook or bake, you can easily substitute two egg whites for one whole egg. That way you lose the fat but keep the recipe the same.

Nuts, peanut butter, and regular cheese are high-fat choices; that's why they're in the outer rings of the Target. More than 70 percent of their total calories comes from fat! These are choices that need to be tracked carefully. You can pick them—but when you do, the fat adds up quickly.

Each of the remaining foods on the Target—**salad dressing, margarine, butter, and oil**—are almost all fat. In fact, oil of any kind is 100 percent fat. When you choose any of these, your fat choices for the day will be used up quickly.

JUST REMEMBER

Foods near the center of the Fat Attack Target have no limits to their use, because they're fat free. But foods in the outer rings of the Target have fat; if you choose them, you need to keep track of it.

Naturally, we wouldn't be talking so much about tracking fat if it weren't important. And it *is* very important to keep track of the fat you eat. But there's more to healthy eating than tracking fat. You depend on the food you eat to supply the raw materials to keep your body strong and healthy. In order to stay well, you need a variety of foods that offer vitamins, minerals, fiber, and protein.

That's why selecting your foods with the help of the Fat Attack Target and planning your daily menus around the food groups in the In Control Menu Planner is the best route to follow. Although you're free to choose any food now that you're In Control, these are things that will help remind you of the most healthy choices.

Sample Days When You're In Control

On pages 248–63 you'll find examples of how you can plan your day's eating so that it keeps you slim and healthy and fits into the way you live. We've worked in typical food choices for each of the sample days and then we've organized *all* that day's foods onto a worksheet showing which food groups the choices fall into. This is a great way to look at a typical day of eating and then to see exactly what you're getting for the food you choose. You can see how much fat there is in all of these choices at a glance, too.

While all these sample days are based on the healthy Menu Planner that we recommend for eating In Control, they include a variety of fat foods. No food choices are "off limits" when you're In Control! With correct planning, it's possible to do just about anything, within reasonable limits.

When you're planning to eat a fast-food dinner, for example, just plan ahead. To show you how easy that is to do, we've put together a "Fast-Food Dinner Day" for you. It shows a low-fat breakfast and lunch, leaving most of the fat choices for dining out. Just be sure to track your fat even more carefully on a day that you're eating fast food.

You can even enjoy a Sunday brunch, complete with omelet, sausage, and a scone, so we've created a "Sunday Brunch Day" to show you how to do just that. On a day like this, have low-fat snacks and a low-fat Sunday supper.

Study these sample days carefully and then think about how you'd put together a typical day of your own. Play around with different foods, checking them out on the Fat-Free Foods list on pages 294–99 and with the help of the Fat Counter, beginning on pages 300. Remember that you don't need to feel locked into a traditional three-meals-a-day pattern. Now that you're In Control, planning what you eat each day is up to you.

And we've made it even easier by giving you several blank In Control Menu Planners to fill in with your favorite foods. For each Menu Planner, there's also a Menu Worksheet that shows the five food groups around which you should be building your day's eating, and it provides space for you to track the fat in the fat-food choices you make. It's a good idea to make even more copies of these Menu Planners and Worksheets to use for as long as you formally track your fat when you're In Control.

Soon you'll have such a good idea of how to keep within your recommended limit that you won't need to use a worksheet and will probably be making your choices using only the Fat Attack Target. And in time you won't even need to look at the target, either—prioritizing your foods will be second nature.

To help you along even more, chapters 10, 11, and 12 offer Fat Attack advice for smart supermarket shopping, creative low-fat cooking, and enjoyable eating out. Before you know it, you'll be able to put yourself on "automatic pilot." Then you'll know you're really In Control!

In Control
MENUS AND
WORKSHEETS

On the following pages you'll find several menu ideas for delicious eating while you're In Control, including suggested portion sizes that will help both men and women keep their daily fat intake within the In Control guidelines. Each Menu Sample is followed by a Menu Worksheet that puts each day's suggested foods into the correct food group.

These are only samples, however; don't feel tied to these particular meal suggestions or to any other specific meal pattern. Remember, when you're In Control *you* decide when and how much you eat. Have three meals and two snacks a day if you want to, but there's no need to feel locked into a traditional eating pattern. If, for example, you'd prefer to have several "mini-meals" throughout the day, go right ahead. Just be sure you're eating lots of nutritious, low-fat foods. And don't forget to track your fat: No more than forty-five grams a day if you're a woman, or sixty grams a day if you're a man.

To help make nutritious meal planning easier during your first weeks In Control, you'll also find fourteen blank Menu Planners and fourteen blank Menu Worksheets. Now that you're making all your own food choices, you'll find these helpful for planning meals based on the five food groups, recording your food choices, and tracking your fat. Of course, if you still want to formally track your fat after the first two weeks, you can use these sheets for as long as you like.

In Control
MENU SAMPLE—DAY 1—WOMEN

BREAKFAST
Orange Sections
1 Bran Muffin
1 Cup Skim Milk
Coffee

SNACK
Diet Cola

LUNCH
Ham and Cheese Sandwich
  2 Slices Rye Bread
  1 Ounce American Cheese
  2 Ounces Sliced Ham
  Lettuce and Tomato
  1 Tablespoon Russian Dressing
1 Cup Skim Milk

DINNER
4 Ounces Halibut
Brown Rice
Carrots and Peas
Large Mixed Salad
3 Tablespoons Reduced-calorie Italian
  Dressing
1/2 Cup Vanilla Ice Cream

SNACK
Sliced Pineapple

MENU WORKSHEET—DAY 1—WOMEN

Food Group	Food Choice	Fat
VITAMIN-RICH FRUITS AND VEGETABLES 5 a day recommended	*Orange Sections* *Lettuce and Tomato* *Carrots and Peas* *Large Mixed Salad* *Sliced Pineapple*	
FIBER-RICH BREAD, CEREAL, PASTA, BEANS, RICE, AND OTHER GRAINS 3 a day recommended	*2 Slices Rye Bread* *Brown Rice*	
CALCIUM-RICH MILK AND YOGURT 2 a day recommended	*2 Cups Skim Milk*	*trace*
PROTEIN-RICH MEAT, FISH, AND POULTRY 6 ounces a day recommended	*2 Ounces Ham* *4 Ounces Halibut*	*6 grams* *3 grams*
ADDITIONAL FAT CHOICES	*1 Bran Muffin* *1 Ounce American Cheese* *1 Tablespoon Russian Dressing* *3 Tablespoons Reduced-calorie Italian Dressing* *½ Cup Vanilla Ice Cream*	*6 grams* *9 grams* *8 grams* *6 grams* *7 grams*

Keep the day's total at or below: *Today's fat total*   *45 grams*

   45 grams of fat for women

   60 grams of fat for men

In Control
SAMPLE—DAY 2—WOMEN

BREAKFAST
Cantaloupe
1 Slice French Toast
1 Cup 1% Milk
Tea

SNACK
Grapes

LUNCH
Chef Salad
  1 Ounce Swiss Cheese
  1 Ounce Roast Beef
3 Tablespoons Reduced-calorie Russian Dressing
Hard Roll
Mineral Water

DINNER
5 Ounces Boneless Chicken Breast
Tricolor Pasta
1 Teaspoon Diet Margarine
1 Tablespoon Grated Parmesan Cheese
Green Beans
Corn on the Cob
1 Chocolate Cupcake with Chocolate Icing

SNACK
Blueberry Low-fat Yogurt

In Control
MENU WORKSHEET—DAY 2—WOMEN

Food Group	Food Choice	Fat
VITAMIN-RICH FRUITS AND VEGETABLES **5 a day recommended**	Cantaloupe Grapes Lunch Salad Green Beans Corn on the Cob	
FIBER-RICH BREAD, CEREAL, PASTA, BEANS, RICE, AND OTHER GRAINS **3 a day recommended**	Hard Roll Tricolor Pasta	
CALCIUM-RICH MILK AND YOGURT **2 a day recommended**	1 Cup 1% Milk Blueberry Low-fat Yogurt	3 grams 2 grams
PROTEIN-RICH MEAT, FISH, AND POULTRY **6 ounces a day recommended**	1 Ounce Roast Beef 5 Ounces Boneless Chicken Breast	2 grams 5 grams

ADDITIONAL FAT CHOICES	1 Slice French Toast
	1 Ounce Swiss Cheese
	3 Tablespoons Reduced-
	  calorie Russian Dressing
	1 Teaspoon Diet Margarine
	1 Tablespoon Grated
	  Parmesan Cheese
	1 Chocolate Cupcake with
	  Chocolate Icing
		7 grams
		8 grams
		
		6 grams
		2 grams
		
		2 grams
		
		8 grams

Keep the day's total at or below: Today's fat total   45 grams
   45 grams of fat for women
   60 grams of fat for men

In Control
MENU SAMPLE
FAST-FOOD DINNER DAY—Women

BREAKFAST
Grapefruit
Raisin Bran Cereal
1 Cup Skim Milk
Coffee

SNACK
English Muffin
Jelly
Tea

LUNCH
1 Cup Lentil Soup
Tuna Salad Sandwich
2 Slices Whole Wheat Bread
½ Cup Tuna Salad
Lettuce and Tomato
1 Tablespoon Reduced-calorie Russian Dressing
1 Cup Skim Milk

DINNER
Cheeseburger with Lettuce, Tomato, and Fixings
Regular-order French Fries
Diet Cola
Apple
2 Gingersnaps

SNACK
Banana

In Control
MENU WORKSHEET
FAST-FOOD DINNER DAY—WOMEN

Food Group	*Food Choice*	*Fat*
VITAMIN-RICH FRUITS AND VEGETABLES 5 a day recommended	*Grapefruit* *Lettuce and Tomato* *Apple* *Banana*	
FIBER-RICH BREAD, CEREAL, PASTA, BEANS, RICE, AND OTHER GRAINS 3 a day recommended	*Raisin Bran* *English Muffin* *2 Slices Whole Wheat Bread* *Hamburger Roll*	
CALCIUM-RICH MILK AND YOGURT 2 a day recommended	*2 Cups Skim Milk*	
PROTEIN-RICH MEAT, FISH, AND POULTRY 6 ounces a day recommended	*½ Cup Tuna Salad* *Cheeseburger*	*8 grams* *20 grams*
ADDITIONAL FAT CHOICES	*1 Cup Lentil Soup* *1 Tablespoon Reduced- calorie Russian Dressing* *Regular-order French Fries* *2 Gingersnaps*	*2 grams* *1 gram* *12 grams* *2 grams*

Keep the day's total at or below: *Today's fat total*   *45 grams*
    45 grams of fat for women
    60 grams of fat for men

In Control
MENU SAMPLE
SUNDAY BRUNCH DAY—WOMEN

BREAKFAST
Strawberries
2-Egg Omelet
2 Smoked Breakfast Sausages
1 Scone
Peach Butter
1 Cup Skim Milk
Coffee

SNACK
Cherries

DINNER
4 Ounces Turkey Breast
Baked Sweet Potato
Asparagus
Oatmeal Bread
Large Mixed Salad
1 Tablespoon French Dressing
½ Cup Pumpkin Pudding
Iced Tea

SNACK
1 Cup Skim Milk
2 Slices Toast

In Control
MENU WORKSHEET
SUNDAY BRUNCH DAY—WOMEN

Food Group	Food Choice	Fat
VITAMIN-RICH FRUITS AND VEGETABLES **5 a day recommended**	*Strawberries* *Cherries* *Sweet Potato* *Asparagus* *Large Mixed Salad*	
FIBER-RICH BREAD, CEREAL, PASTA, BEANS, RICE, AND OTHER GRAINS **3 a day recommended**	*1 Slice Oatmeal Bread* *2 Slices Toast*	
CALCIUM-RICH MILK AND YOGURT **2 a day recommended**	*2 Cups Skim Milk*	
PROTEIN-RICH MEAT, FISH, AND POULTRY **6 ounces a day recommended**	*2-Egg Omelet* *4 Ounces Turkey Breast*	*14 grams* *3 grams*
ADDITIONAL FAT CHOICES	*2 Sausages* *1 Scone* *1 Tablespoon French Dressing* *½ Cup Pumpkin Pudding*	*10 grams* *6 grams* *6 grams* *5 grams*

Keep the day's total at or below: *Today's fat total*   *44 grams*
   45 grams of fat for women
   60 grams of fat for men

In Control
MENU SAMPLE—DAY 1—MEN

BREAKFAST
Orange Sections
1 Bran Muffin
1 Cup Skim Milk
Coffee

SNACK
Bagel
1 Ounce Cream Cheese
Tea

LUNCH
Ham and Cheese Club Sandwich
  3 Slices Rye Bread
  1 Ounce American Cheese
  2 Ounces Sliced Ham
  Lettuce and Tomato
  1 Tablespoon Russian Dressing
1 Cup Skim Milk

DINNER
4 Ounces Halibut
Brown Rice
Carrots and Peas
Large Mixed Salad
3 Tablespoons Reduced-calorie Italian
  Dressing
¾ Cup Vanilla Ice Cream

SNACK
Sliced Pineapple

In Control
MENU WORKSHEET—DAY 1—MEN

Food Group	Food Choice	Fat
VITAMIN-RICH FRUITS AND VEGETABLES **5 a day recommended**	*Orange Sections* *Lettuce and Tomato* *Carrots and Peas* *Large Mixed Salad* *Sliced Pineapple*	
FIBER-RICH BREAD, CEREAL, PASTA, BEANS, RICE, AND OTHER GRAINS **3 a day recommended**	*1 Bagel* *3 Slices Rye Bread* *Brown Rice*	
CALCIUM-RICH MILK AND YOGURT **2 a day recommended**	*2 Cups Skim Milk*	*trace*
PROTEIN-RICH MEAT, FISH, AND POULTRY **6 ounces a day recommended**	*2 Ounces Ham* *4 Ounces Halibut*	*6 grams* *3 grams*
ADDITIONAL FAT CHOICES	*1 Bran Muffin* *1 Ounce Cream Cheese* *1 Ounce American Cheese* *1 Tablespoon Russian Dressing* *3 Tablespoons Reduced-calorie Italian Dressing* *¾ Cup Vanilla Ice Cream*	*6 grams* *10 grams* *9 grams* *8 grams* *6 grams* *11 grams*

Keep the day's total at or below: *Today's fat total*   59 grams
   45 grams of fat for women
   60 grams of fat for men

In Control
MENU SAMPLE—DAY 2—MEN

BREAKFAST
Cantaloupe
2 Slices French Toast
1 Cup 1% Milk
Tea

SNACK
Grapes

LUNCH
Chef Salad
   1 Ounce Ham
   1 Ounce Swiss Cheese
   1 Ounce Roast Beef
4 Tablespoons Reduced-calorie Russian Dressing
Hard Roll
Mineral Water

DINNER
5-Ounce Boneless Chicken Breast
Tricolor Pasta
1 Teaspoon Margarine
1 Tablespoon Grated Parmesan Cheese
Green Beans
Corn on the Cob
1 Chocolate Cupcake with Chocolate Icing

SNACK
1 Cup Blueberry Low-fat Yogurt

In Control
MENU WORKSHEET—DAY 2—MEN

Food Group	Food Choice	Fat
VITAMIN-RICH FRUITS AND VEGETABLES 5 a day recommended	Cantaloupe Grapes Lunch Salad Green Beans Corn on the Cob	
FIBER-RICH BREAD, CEREAL, PASTA, BEANS, RICE, AND OTHER GRAINS 3 a day recommended	Hard Roll Tricolor Pasta	
CALCIUM-RICH MILK AND YOGURT 2 a day recommended	1 Cup 1% Milk 1 Cup Blueberry Low-fat Yogurt	3 grams 2 grams
PROTEIN-RICH MEAT, FISH, AND POULTRY 6 ounces a day recommended	1 Ounce Roast Beef 1 Ounce Ham 5 Ounces Boneless Chicken Breast	2 grams 3 grams 5 grams
ADDITIONAL FAT CHOICES	2 Slices French Toast 1 Ounce Swiss Cheese 4 Tablespoons Reduced- calorie Russian Dressing 1 Teaspoon Margarine 1 Tablespoon Grated Parmesan Cheese 1 Chocolate Cupcake with Chocolate Icing	14 grams 8 grams 8 grams 4 grams 2 grams 8 grams

Keep the day's total at or below: Today's fat total   59 grams
    45 grams of fat for women
    60 grams of fat for men

In Control
MENU SAMPLE
FAST-FOOD DINNER DAY—MEN

BREAKFAST
Grapefruit
Raisin Bran Cereal
1 Cup Skim Milk
Coffee

SNACK
English Muffin
Jelly
Tea

LUNCH
1 Cup Lentil Soup
Tuna Salad Sandwich
   2 Slices Whole Wheat Bread
   1/2 Cup Tuna Salad
Lettuce and Tomato
1 Tablespoon Reduced-calorie Russian
Dressing
1 Cup Skim Milk

DINNER
Double Cheeseburger with Lettuce, Tomato,
   and Fixings
Regular-order French Fries
Diet Cola
Apple
2 Gingersnaps

SNACK
Banana

In Control
MENU WORKSHEET
FAST-FOOD DINNER DAY—MEN

Food Group	*Food Choice*	*Fat*
VITAMIN-RICH FRUITS AND VEGETABLES 5 a day recommended	*Grapefruit* *Lettuce and Tomato* *Apple* *Banana*	
FIBER-RICH BREAD, CEREAL, PASTA, BEANS, RICE, AND OTHER GRAINS 3 a day recommended	*Raisin Bran* *English Muffin* *2 Slices Whole Wheat Bread* *Hamburger Roll*	
CALCIUM-RICH MILK AND YOGURT 2 a day recommended	*2 Cups Skim Milk*	
PROTEIN-RICH MEAT, FISH, AND POULTRY 6 ounces a day recommended	*½ Cup Tuna Salad* *Double Cheeseburger*	*8 grams* *35 grams*
ADDITIONAL FAT CHOICES	*1 Cup Lentil Soup* *1 Tablespoon Reduced-calorie Russian Dressing* *Regular-order French Fries* *2 Gingersnaps*	*2 grams* *1 gram* *12 grams* *2 grams*

Keep the day's total at or below: *Today's fat total*   60 grams
   45 grams of fat for women
   60 grams of fat for men

In Control
MENU SAMPLE
SUNDAY BRUNCH DAY—MEN

BREAKFAST
Strawberries
2-Egg Omelet
2 Smoked Breakfast Sausages
1 Scone
Peach Butter
1 Cup Skim Milk
Coffee

SNACK
Cherries

DINNER
4 Ounces Turkey Breast
Baked Sweet Potato
Asparagus
Oatmeal Bread
2 Teaspoons Margarine
Large Mixed Salad
2 Tablespoons French Dressing
1/2 Cup Pumpkin Pudding
Iced Tea

SNACK
1 Cup Skim Milk
2 Slices Toast

In Control
MENU WORKSHEET
SUNDAY BRUNCH DAY—MEN

Food Group	Food Choice	Fat
VITAMIN-RICH FRUITS AND VEGETABLES 5 a day recommended	*Strawberries* *Cherries* *Sweet Potato* *Asparagus* *Large Mixed Salad*	
FIBER-RICH BREAD, CEREAL, PASTA, BEANS, RICE, AND OTHER GRAINS 3 a day recommended	*1 Slice Oatmeal Bread* *2 Slices Toast*	
CALCIUM-RICH MILK AND YOGURT 2 a day recommended	*2 Cups Skim Milk*	
PROTEIN-RICH MEAT, FISH, AND POULTRY 6 ounces a day recommended	*2-Egg Omelet* *4 Ounces Turkey Breast*	*14 grams* *3 grams*
ADDITIONAL FAT CHOICES	*2 Sausages* *1 Scone* *2 Tablespoons French Dressing* *2 Teaspoons Margarine* *½ Cup Pumpkin Pudding*	*10 grams* *6 grams* *12 grams* *8 grams* *5 grams*
Keep the day's total at or below:	*Today's fat total*	*58 grams*

    45 grams of fat for women
    60 grams of fat for men

In Control
MENU PLANNER

BREAKFAST

_____

_____

_____

_____

_____

_____

SNACK

_____

LUNCH

_____

_____

_____

_____

DINNER

_____

_____

_____

_____

_____

SNACK

_____

Although the In Control Menu Worksheet has been set up with room for Breakfast, Lunch, Dinner, and Snack entries, there's no need to feel locked into a traditional eating pattern. Rather, when you're In Control, you make all the decisions about what—and when—you eat. If, for example, you'd prefer to have several "mini-meals" throughout the day, go right ahead. As long as you track your fat and keep it within the 45/60-gram guidelines, the size and timing of your meals are up to you.

In Control
MENU WORKSHEET

Food Group	Food Choice	Fat Grams
VITAMIN-RICH FRUITS AND VEGETABLES 5 a day recommended	_____ _____ _____ _____ _____	
FIBER-RICH BREAD, CEREAL, PASTA, BEANS, RICE, AND OTHER GRAINS 3 a day recommended	_____ _____ _____	
CALCIUM-RICH MILK AND YOGURT 2 a day recommended	_____ _____	_____ _____
PROTEIN-RICH MEAT, FISH, AND POULTRY 6 ounces a day recommended	_____ _____ _____ _____ _____ _____ _____	_____ _____ _____ _____ _____ _____ _____
ADDITIONAL FAT CHOICES	_____ _____ _____ _____	_____ _____ _____ _____

Keep the day's total at or below: *Today's Fat Total* _____
   45 grams of fat for women
   60 grams of fat for men

In Control
MENU PLANNER

BREAKFAST

_____
_____
_____
_____
_____
_____

SNACK

_____
_____

LUNCH

_____
_____
_____
_____
_____

DINNER

_____
_____
_____
_____
_____

SNACK

_____
_____

In Control
MENU WORKSHEET

Food Group	Food Choice	Fat Grams
VITAMIN-RICH FRUITS AND VEGETABLES 5 a day recommended	_____ _____ _____ _____ _____	
FIBER-RICH BREAD, CEREAL, PASTA, BEANS, RICE, AND OTHER GRAINS 3 a day recommended	_____ _____ _____	
CALCIUM-RICH MILK AND YOGURT 2 a day recommended	_____ _____	_____ _____
PROTEIN-RICH MEAT, FISH, AND POULTRY 6 ounces a day recommended	_____ _____ _____ _____ _____ _____	_____ _____ _____ _____ _____ _____
ADDITIONAL FAT CHOICES	_____ _____ _____ _____	_____ _____ _____ _____

Keep the day's total at or below: *Today's Fat Total* _____
   45 grams of fat for women
   60 grams of fat for men

In Control
MENU PLANNER

BREAKFAST

_____
_____
_____
_____
_____
_____

SNACK

_____
_____

LUNCH

_____
_____
_____
_____

DINNER

_____
_____
_____
_____
_____

SNACK

_____
_____

In Control
MENU WORKSHEET

Food Group	Food Choice	Fat Grams
VITAMIN-RICH FRUITS AND VEGETABLES 5 a day recommended	_____ _____ _____ _____ _____	
FIBER-RICH BREAD, CEREAL, PASTA, BEANS, RICE, AND OTHER GRAINS 3 a day recommended	_____ _____ _____	
CALCIUM-RICH MILK AND YOGURT 2 a day recommended	_____ _____	_____ _____
PROTEIN-RICH MEAT, FISH, AND POULTRY 6 ounces a day recommended	_____ _____ _____ _____ _____ _____	_____ _____ _____ _____ _____ _____
ADDITIONAL FAT CHOICES	_____ _____ _____ _____	_____ _____ _____ _____

Keep the day's total at or below: *Today's Fat Total* _____
   45 grams of fat for women
   60 grams of fat for men

In Control
MENU PLANNER

BREAKFAST

_____
_____
_____
_____
_____
_____

SNACK

_____
_____

LUNCH

_____
_____
_____
_____
_____

DINNER

_____
_____
_____
_____
_____
_____

SNACK

_____
_____

In Control
MENU WORKSHEET

Food Group	Food Choice	Fat Grams
VITAMIN-RICH FRUITS AND VEGETABLES 5 a day recommended	_____ _____ _____ _____ _____	
FIBER-RICH BREAD, CEREAL, PASTA, BEANS, RICE, AND OTHER GRAINS 3 a day recommended	_____ _____ _____	
CALCIUM-RICH MILK AND YOGURT 2 a day recommended	_____ _____	_____ _____
PROTEIN-RICH MEAT, FISH, AND POULTRY 6 ounces a day recommended	_____ _____ _____ _____ _____ _____	_____ _____ _____ _____ _____ _____
ADDITIONAL FAT CHOICES	_____ _____ _____ _____	_____ _____ _____ _____

Keep the day's total at or below: *Today's Fat Total* _____
   45 grams of fat for women
   60 grams of fat for men

In Control
MENU PLANNER

BREAKFAST

_____
_____
_____
_____
_____

SNACK

_____
_____

LUNCH

_____
_____
_____
_____
_____

DINNER

_____
_____
_____
_____
_____

SNACK

_____
_____

In Control
MENU WORKSHEET

Food Group	Food Choice	Fat Grams
VITAMIN-RICH FRUITS AND VEGETABLES 5 a day recommended	_____ _____ _____ _____ _____	
FIBER-RICH BREAD, CEREAL, PASTA, BEANS, RICE, AND OTHER GRAINS 3 a day recommended	_____ _____ _____	
CALCIUM-RICH MILK AND YOGURT 2 a day recommended	_____ _____	_____ _____
PROTEIN-RICH MEAT, FISH, AND POULTRY 6 ounces a day recommended	_____ _____ _____ _____ _____ _____	_____ _____ _____ _____ _____ _____
ADDITIONAL FAT CHOICES	_____ _____ _____ _____	_____ _____ _____ _____

Keep the day's total at or below: *Today's Fat Total* _____

    45 grams of fat for women

    60 grams of fat for men

In Control
MENU PLANNER

BREAKFAST

_____
_____
_____
_____
_____

SNACK

_____
_____

LUNCH

_____
_____
_____
_____

DINNER

_____
_____
_____
_____
_____

SNACK

_____
_____

In Control
MENU WORKSHEET

Food Group	Food Choice	Fat Grams
VITAMIN-RICH FRUITS AND VEGETABLES 5 a day recommended	_____	
	_____	
	_____	
	_____	
	_____	
FIBER-RICH BREAD, CEREAL, PASTA, BEANS, RICE, AND OTHER GRAINS 3 a day recommended	_____	
	_____	
	_____	
CALCIUM-RICH MILK AND YOGURT 2 a day recommended	_____	_____
	_____	_____
PROTEIN-RICH MEAT, FISH, AND POULTRY 6 ounces a day recommended	_____	_____
	_____	_____
	_____	_____
	_____	_____
	_____	_____
ADDITIONAL FAT CHOICES	_____	_____
	_____	_____
	_____	_____
	_____	_____

Keep the day's total at or below: *Today's Fat Total* _____
   45 grams of fat for women
   60 grams of fat for men

In Control
MENU PLANNER

BREAKFAST

_____
_____
_____
_____
_____
_____

SNACK

_____
_____

LUNCH

_____
_____
_____
_____
_____

DINNER

_____
_____
_____
_____
_____
_____

SNACK

_____
_____

In Control
MENU WORKSHEET

Food Group	Food Choice	Fat Grams
VITAMIN-RICH FRUITS AND VEGETABLES 5 a day recommended	_____ _____ _____ _____ _____	
FIBER-RICH BREAD, CEREAL, PASTA, BEANS, RICE, AND OTHER GRAINS 3 a day recommended	_____ _____ _____	
CALCIUM-RICH MILK AND YOGURT 2 a day recommended	_____ _____	_____ _____
PROTEIN-RICH MEAT, FISH, AND POULTRY 6 ounces a day recommended	_____ _____ _____ _____ _____ _____	_____ _____ _____ _____ _____ _____
ADDITIONAL FAT CHOICES	_____ _____ _____ _____	_____ _____ _____ _____

Keep the day's total at or below: *Today's Fat Total* _____
  45 grams of fat for women
  60 grams of fat for men

In Control
MENU PLANNER

BREAKFAST

_____

_____

_____

_____

_____

_____

SNACK

_____

_____

LUNCH

_____

_____

_____

_____

_____

DINNER

_____

_____

_____

_____

_____

_____

SNACK

_____

_____

In Control
MENU WORKSHEET

Food Group	Food Choice	Fat Grams
VITAMIN-RICH FRUITS AND VEGETABLES 5 a day recommended	_____ _____ _____ _____ _____	
FIBER-RICH BREAD, CEREAL, PASTA, BEANS, RICE, AND OTHER GRAINS 3 a day recommended	_____ _____ _____	
CALCIUM-RICH MILK AND YOGURT 2 a day recommended	_____ _____	_____ _____
PROTEIN-RICH MEAT, FISH, AND POULTRY 6 ounces a day recommended	_____ _____ _____ _____ _____ _____	_____ _____ _____ _____ _____ _____
ADDITIONAL FAT CHOICES	_____ _____ _____ _____	_____ _____ _____ _____

Keep the day's total at or below: *Today's Fat Total* _____
    45 grams of fat for women
    60 grams of fat for men

In Control
MENU PLANNER

BREAKFAST

_____

_____

_____

_____

_____

_____

SNACK

_____

_____

LUNCH

_____

_____

_____

_____

_____

DINNER

_____

_____

_____

_____

_____

_____

SNACK

_____

_____

In Control
MENU WORKSHEET

Food Group	Food Choice	Fat Grams
VITAMIN-RICH FRUITS AND VEGETABLES 5 a day recommended	_____ _____ _____ _____ _____	
FIBER-RICH BREAD, CEREAL, PASTA, BEANS, RICE, AND OTHER GRAINS 3 a day recommended	_____ _____ _____	
CALCIUM-RICH MILK AND YOGURT 2 a day recommended	_____ _____	_____ _____
PROTEIN-RICH MEAT, FISH, AND POULTRY 6 ounces a day recommended	_____ _____ _____ _____ _____	_____ _____ _____ _____ _____
ADDITIONAL FAT CHOICES	_____ _____ _____ _____	_____ _____ _____ _____

Keep the day's total at or below:
   45 grams of fat for women
   60 grams of fat for men

Today's Fat Total _____

In Control
MENU PLANNER

BREAKFAST

_____
_____
_____
_____
_____
_____

SNACK

_____
_____

LUNCH

_____
_____
_____
_____
_____

DINNER

_____
_____
_____
_____
_____
_____

SNACK

_____
_____

In Control
MENU WORKSHEET

Food Group	Food Choice	Fat Grams
VITAMIN-RICH FRUITS AND VEGETABLES 5 a day recommended	_____	
	_____	
	_____	
	_____	
	_____	
FIBER-RICH BREAD, CEREAL, PASTA, BEANS, RICE, AND OTHER GRAINS 3 a day recommended	_____	
	_____	
	_____	
CALCIUM-RICH MILK AND YOGURT 2 a day recommended	_____	_____
	_____	_____
PROTEIN-RICH MEAT, FISH, AND POULTRY 6 ounces a day recommended	_____	_____
	_____	_____
	_____	_____
	_____	_____
	_____	_____
ADDITIONAL FAT CHOICES	_____	_____
	_____	_____
	_____	_____
	_____	_____

Keep the day's total at or below: *Today's Fat Total* _____
   45 grams of fat for women
   60 grams of fat for men

In Control
MENU PLANNER

BREAKFAST

_____
_____
_____
_____
_____
_____

SNACK

_____
_____

LUNCH

_____
_____
_____
_____
_____

DINNER

_____
_____
_____
_____
_____

SNACK

_____
_____

In Control
MENU WORKSHEET

Food Group	Food Choice	Fat Grams
VITAMIN-RICH FRUITS AND VEGETABLES 5 a day recommended	_____	
	_____	
	_____	
	_____	
	_____	
FIBER-RICH BREAD, CEREAL, PASTA, BEANS, RICE, AND OTHER GRAINS 3 a day recommended	_____	
	_____	
	_____	
CALCIUM-RICH MILK AND YOGURT 2 a day recommended	_____	_____
	_____	_____
PROTEIN-RICH MEAT, FISH, AND POULTRY 6 ounces a day recommended	_____	_____
	_____	_____
	_____	_____
	_____	_____
	_____	_____
ADDITIONAL FAT CHOICES	_____	_____
	_____	_____
	_____	_____
	_____	_____

Keep the day's total at or below:
   45 grams of fat for women
   60 grams of fat for men

Today's Fat Total _____

In Control
MENU PLANNER

BREAKFAST

_____
_____
_____
_____
_____

SNACK

_____
_____

LUNCH

_____
_____
_____
_____

DINNER

_____
_____
_____
_____
_____

SNACK

_____
_____

In Control
MENU WORKSHEET

Food Group	Food Choice	Fat Grams
VITAMIN-RICH FRUITS AND VEGETABLES 5 a day recommended	_____ _____ _____ _____ _____	
FIBER-RICH BREAD, CEREAL, PASTA, BEANS, RICE, AND OTHER GRAINS 3 a day recommended	_____ _____ _____	
CALCIUM-RICH MILK AND YOGURT 2 a day recommended	_____ _____	_____ _____
PROTEIN-RICH MEAT, FISH, AND POULTRY 6 ounces a day recommended	_____ _____ _____ _____ _____ _____	_____ _____ _____ _____ _____ _____
ADDITIONAL FAT CHOICES	_____ _____ _____ _____	_____ _____ _____ _____

Keep the day's total at or below: Today's Fat Total   _____
   45 grams of fat for women
   60 grams of fat for men

In Control
MENU PLANNER

BREAKFAST

_____
_____
_____
_____
_____
_____

SNACK

_____
_____

LUNCH

_____
_____
_____
_____
_____

DINNER

_____
_____
_____
_____
_____

SNACK

_____
_____

In Control
MENU WORKSHEET

Food Group	Food Choice	Fat Grams
VITAMIN-RICH FRUITS AND VEGETABLES 5 a day recommended	_____	
	_____	
	_____	
	_____	
	_____	
FIBER-RICH BREAD, CEREAL, PASTA, BEANS, RICE, AND OTHER GRAINS 3 a day recommended	_____	
	_____	
	_____	
CALCIUM-RICH MILK AND YOGURT 2 a day recommended	_____	_____
	_____	_____
PROTEIN-RICH MEAT, FISH, AND POULTRY 6 ounces a day recommended	_____	_____
	_____	_____
	_____	_____
	_____	_____
	_____	_____
ADDITIONAL FAT CHOICES	_____	_____
	_____	_____
	_____	_____
	_____	_____

Keep the day's total at or below: *Today's Fat Total*   _____
    45 grams of fat for women
    60 grams of fat for men

In Control
MENU PLANNER

BREAKFAST

_____
_____
_____
_____
_____
_____

SNACK

_____
_____

LUNCH

_____
_____
_____
_____
_____

DINNER

_____
_____
_____
_____
_____
_____

SNACK

_____
_____

In Control
MENU WORKSHEET

Food Group	Food Choice	Fat Grams
VITAMIN-RICH FRUITS AND VEGETABLES 5 a day recommended	_____	
FIBER-RICH BREAD, CEREAL, PASTA, BEANS, RICE, AND OTHER GRAINS 3 a day recommended	_____	
CALCIUM-RICH MILK AND YOGURT 2 a day recommended	_____	_____
PROTEIN-RICH MEAT, FISH, AND POULTRY 6 ounces a day recommended	_____	_____
ADDITIONAL FAT CHOICES	_____	_____

Keep the day's total at or below: *Today's Fat Total* _____
   45 grams of fat for women
   60 grams of fat for men

In Control
FOOD LISTS

These lists make it easier for you to attack your fat when you're In Control. Refer to them whenever you're choosing a food.

You may eat as much of the foods on the **Fat-Free Foods** list as you wish. Fat-free foods are "free" when you're In Control, and because they contain no fat they don't need to be tracked.

If you're choosing a fat food, track the fat in it by referring to the **Fat Counter**, which lists almost one thousand different foods containing fat.

During In Control, use:

      Fat-Free Foods
      Fat Attack Plan Fat Counter

In Control FAT-FREE FOODS

*All of these foods have very little or no fat, provided they are fresh, or packaged, or prepared without added fat. **You do not have to track the fat in these foods to stay IN CONTROL.***

Acerola cherries
Adzuki beans
Ale
Alfalfa sprouts
Amaranth, cooked
Apple
  canned
  dried
  fresh
  juice
Apricot
  canned
  dried
  fresh
Arrowhead
Artichoke
  canned
  fresh
  frozen
Asparagus
  canned
  fresh
  frozen
Bagel
Bamboo shoots
Banana
Beans
  canned
  dried
  frozen
  sprouts
Beer
Beets
  canned
  fresh

Blackberries
  canned
  fresh
  frozen
Black-eyed peas
  canned
  dried
  frozen
Blueberries
  canned
  fresh
  frozen
Borage
Boysenberries
  canned
  fresh
  juice
Bread
  bran
  brown bread, canned
  cracked wheat
  French
  Italian
  multigrain
  oat
  pumpernickel
  raisin
  rye
  wheat berry
  white
  whole wheat
Breadfruit
Breadsticks
Broad beans
  canned

dried
fresh
Broccoli
  fresh
  frozen
Brussels sprouts
  fresh
  frozen
Bulgur
Burdock root
Butter beans
  canned
  dried
Butter sprinkles
Cabbage
  canned
  fresh
Cake
  angel food
Candy
  gumdrops
  gummy shapes
  hard candy
  jelly beans
  licorice
  lollipops
Cantaloupe
Carambola
Cardoon
Carob flour
Carrot
  canned
  fresh
  frozen
  juice
Casaba
Cauliflower
  fresh
  frozen
Celeriac

Celery
Celtuce
Chayote
Cherries
  candied
  canned
  fresh
  frozen
  juice
Chestnuts
Chick-peas
  canned
  dried
Chicory
Chives
Citron
Coffee
  decaffeinated
  instant
  regular
Coffee substitutes
Collards
  fresh
  frozen
Corn
  canned
  fresh
  frozen
Cornmeal
Cornstarch
Cowpeas
  canned
  dried
  frozen
Crabapple
Cranberries
  canned
  fresh
  juice
Cranberry beans

In Control FAT-FREE FOODS (*cont.*)

canned
dried
Cress
Cucumber
Currants
Dandelion greens
Dates
Dock
Eggplant
Elderberries
Endive
English muffin
Figs
  canned
  dried
  fresh
Flour
  bread
  high protein
  potato
  rice
  rye
  unbleached
  white
  whole wheat
French beans
Fructose
Fruit cocktail
Fruit salad
Garlic
Gelatin
  drinks
  mix
Ginkgo nuts
Gooseberries
  canned
  fresh
Grapes

canned
fresh
juice
Grapefruit
  canned
  fresh
  juice
Great northern beans
  canned
  dried
Green beans
  canned
  fresh
  frozen
Ground-cherries
Guava
Herbs
  fresh
  dried
Honeydew
Horseradish
Hyacinth beans
Ice pops, fruit or fruit juice only
Italian ice, all flavors
Jam, all varieties
Jelly, all varieties
Kale
  fresh
  frozen
Ketchup
Kidney beans
  canned
  dried
  sprouts
Kiwi
Kohlrabi
Kumquats
Lamb's-quarters

Leeks
  dried
  fresh
Lemon
  candied
  fresh
  juice
Lentils
  canned
  dried
  sprouts
Lettuce, all varieties
Lima beans
  canned
  dried
  fresh
  frozen
Lime
  fresh
  juice
Liquor/liqueur, all varieties
Loganberries
Loquats
Lotus root
Mango
Marshmallow
Matzo
Mineral water, all varieties
Molasses
Mung beans
  dried
  sprouts
Mushrooms
  canned
  dried
  fresh
Mustard, all varieties
Mustard greens
  fresh
  frozen

Natto
Navy beans
  canned
  dried
  sprouts
Nectarine
Okra
  canned
  fresh
  frozen
Onion
  canned
  dried
  fresh
  frozen
Orange
  candied
  canned
  fresh
  juice
Pancake/waffle syrup
Papaya
Parsnip
Passion fruit
Pasta, all shapes
  regular
  spinach
  tricolor
  whole wheat
Peach
  canned
  dried
  fresh
  frozen
  juice
Pear
  canned
  dried
  fresh
  juice

Peas
  canned
  dried
  fresh
  frozen
Pectin
Pepper
  canned
  dried
  fresh
  frozen
Persimmon
Pickles
Pigeon peas
Pimiento
Pineapple
  candied
  canned
  dried
  fresh
  frozen
  juice
Pink beans
Pinto beans
  canned
  dried
  frozen
  sprouts
Plantains
Plum
  canned
  fresh
Poi
Pokeberry shoots
Pomegranate
Popcorn, air-popped
Potato
  canned

fresh
Potato starch
Pretzels
  regular
  unsalted
  whole wheat
Prunes
  canned
  dried
  juice
Pumpkin
  canned
  fresh
Purslane
Radish
  dried
  fresh
Raisins
Raspberries
  canned
  fresh
  frozen
  juice
Rhubarb
Rice
  bran
  brown
  white
  wild
Rice cakes
Rutabaga
Salsify
Salt/seasoned salt
Salt substitute
Sauerkraut
  canned
  juice
Shallot

Shellie beans
Snap beans
  canned
  fresh
  frozen
Soda, all flavors
  regular
  diet
Sorbet
Soy sauce
Spices
Spinach
  canned
  fresh
  frozen
Squash, all varieties
  canned
  fresh
  frozen
Strawberries
  fresh
  frozen
  juice
Sugar
  brown
  cube
  powder
  raw
  white
Sugar substitutes
Sweet potato
  canned
  fresh
  frozen
Tamarind
Tangerine
  fresh

frozen
Tea
  decaffeinated
  herbal
  instant
  regular
Tomato
  canned
  dried
  fresh
  juice
Turnip
  canned
  fresh
  frozen
Vinegar, all flavors
Water chestnuts
Watercress
Watermelon
Wax beans
White beans
  canned
  dried
Wine, all flavors
Wine coolers
Winged peas
Yam
  canned
  fresh
  frozen
Yard-long beans
Yeast
Zucchini
  canned
  fresh
  frozen

The Fat Attack Plan FAT COUNTER

All of these foods contain fat; tr (trace) indicates fat content of less than 1 gram. Track the fat in these foods when you are In Control.

Food	Serving Size	Fat Grams
Abalone		
fried	3 ounces	6
raw	3 ounces	1
Almonds		
almond butter	1 tablespoon	10
almond paste	1 ounce	8
dry roasted	1 ounce	15
oil roasted	1 ounce	16
toasted	1 ounce	14
Anchovy, canned in oil	1 can (1.6 ounces)	4
Artichoke hearts, canned, marinated	3.5 ounces	26
Avocado	1	31
Bacon		
bacon substitute	1 strip	2
Canadian bacon; grilled	2 slices (1.7 ounces)	4
cooked	3 strips	9
Bass; cooked	3 ounces	2
Beans		
baked beans with beef	½ cup	5
baked beans with franks	½ cup	8
baked beans with pork	½ cup	2
refried beans	½ cup	2
three-bean salad	¾ cup	11
Beef		
bottom round, lean only; braised	3 ounces	8
brisket, whole, lean only; braised	3 ounces	11
cheeseburger with bun	1	15
cheeseburger with bun	1 large	33
cheeseburger with bun, ketchup, mustard, pickles, and onions	1	16

cheeseburger with bun, ketchup, mustard, mayonnaise-style dressing, pickles, onions, lettuce, and tomatoes	1	20
cheeseburger with bun, ketchup, mustard, mayonnaise-style dressing, pickles, onions, lettuce, and tomatoes	1 large	30
cheeseburger with bun, ham, ketchup, mustard, mayonnaise-style dressing, pickles, onions, lettuce, and tomatoes	1 large	48
cheeseburger, double meat patty with bun	1	28
cheeseburger, double meat patty with bun, ketchup, mayonnaise-style dressing, pickles, onions, lettuce, and tomatoes	1	21
cheeseburger, double meat patty with bun, ketchup, mayonnaise-style dressing, pickles, onions, lettuce, and tomatoes	1 large	44
cheeseburger, double meat patty with double-decker bun	1	22
cheeseburger, double meat patty with double-decker bun, ketchup, mustard, mayonnaise-style dressing, pickles, onions, lettuce, and tomatoes	1	35
cheeseburger, triple meat patty with bun	1 large	51
chuck arm pot roast, lean only; braised	3 ounces	9
corned beef, canned	1 ounce	4
eye of round, lean only; roasted	3 ounces	6
flank, lean only; braised	3 ounces	12
ground, extra lean; cooked medium	3 ounces	14
ground, lean; cooked medium	3 ounces	16
ground, regular; cooked medium	3 ounces	18
hamburger with bun	1	12

Food	Serving Size	Fat Grams
hamburger with bun	1 large	23
hamburger with bun, ketchup, mustard, pickles, and onions	1	10
hamburger with bun, ketchup, mustard, pickles, and onions	1 small	5
hamburger with bun, ketchup, mustard, pickles, lettuce, and tomatoes	1 large	13
hamburger, double meat patty with bun	1	28
hamburger, double meat patty with bun, ketchup, mustard, pickles, and onions	1	33
hamburger, triple meat patty with bun, ketchup, mustard, pickles, and onions	1	41
porterhouse steak, lean only; broiled	3 ounces	9
rib, large end, lean only; roasted	3 ounces	12
rib, small end, lean only; roasted	3 ounces	12
rib, whole, lean only; roasted	3 ounces	12
round, lean only; broiled	3 ounces	7
roast beef sandwich	1	14
roast beef sandwich with cheese	1	18
roast beef submarine sandwich with tomato, lettuce, mayonnaise	1	13
shank, crosscut, lean & fat; simmered	3 ounces	10
short ribs, lean & fat; braised	3 ounces	36
sirloin, wedge bone, lean only; broiled	3 ounces	26
steak sandwich	1	14
stroganoff	¾ cup	19
Swiss steak	4.6 ounces	9
T-bone, lean only; broiled	3 ounces	9
tip round, lean only; roasted	3 ounces	7
top round, lean only; broiled	3 ounces	7

Biscuit		
plain	1 (1.5 ounces)	10
plain	1 (2.5 ounces)	13
with egg	1	20
with egg and bacon	1	31
with egg and ham	1	27
with egg and sausage	1	39
with egg and steak	1	28
with egg, cheese, and bacon	1	31
with ham	1	18
with sausage	1	32
with steak	1	26
Blintze, cheese	1	3
Brains		
beef; pan fried	3 ounces	11
pork; braised	3 ounces	8
Brazil Nuts, dried, unblanched	1 ounce	19
Bread		
banana	½" slice	6
corn bread	2" x 2" piece	2
corn stick	1 (1.4 ounces)	4
date-nut	½" slice	3
hush puppies	1 (2 ounces)	7
nut	1 slice (1.5 ounces)	4
pumpkin	1 slice (1.5 ounces)	5
Brownie		
plain	1 (2 ounces)	10
with nuts	1 (.8 ounce)	5
Butter		
regular	1 teaspoon	4
regular	1 pat	4
whipped	1 teaspoon	3
Butternuts, dried	1 ounce	16
Cake		
angel food cake	1/12 cake	tr
apple cake	1.5 ounce piece	7

Food	Serving Size	Fat Grams
baklava	1 ounce	9
boston cream	⅛ of 9" cake	17
carrot with cream cheese	⅟₁₆ cake	21
cheesecake	⅟₁₂ cake	18
chocolate cupcake	1 (1.1 ounces)	5
chocolate cupcake with chocolate icing	1 (1.6 ounces)	8
cobbler, peach	½ cup	6
cream puff with custard filling	1 (4.6 ounces)	18
cream puff, shell only	1 (2.3 ounces)	12
crumb coffee cake	⅛ cake	7
devil's food cake with chocolate frosting	⅟₁₆ cake	8
devil's food cupcake with chocolate frosting	1	4
fruitcake, dark	⅔" slice	7
gingerbread	⅑ cake	4
hot cross bun	1 (1.8 ounces)	7
kuchen	2¼" x 2¼"	13
peanut butter cake	1.8 ounce piece	11
sheet cake with white frosting	⅑ cake	14
sheet cake without frosting	⅑ cake	12
spice cake with caramel icing	⅟₁₀ of 9" cake	16
strudel	4.1 ounce piece	8
toaster pastries	1 (1.9 ounces)	6
torte, chocolate	⅟₁₆ of 8½" diameter	22
white cupcake	1 (1.1 ounces)	5
white cupcake with white icing	1 (1.6 ounces)	6
yellow cake with chocolate icing	⅟₁₆ cake	8
yellow cupcake	1 (1.1 ounces)	5
yellow cupcake with chocolate icing	1 (1.6 ounces)	7
Candy		
caramels	1 ounce	3
chocolate covered raisins	1 ounce	5
fudge, chocolate	1 ounce	3

malted milk balls, chocolate covered	1	2
milk chocolate, plain	1 ounce	9
milk chocolate, with almonds	1 ounce	10
milk chocolate, with peanuts	1 ounce	11
milk chocolate, with rice cereal	1 ounce	7
peanut brittle	1 ounce	3
Carp; cooked	3 ounces	6
Cashews		
cashew butter	1 tablespoon	8
dry roasted	1 ounce	13
oil roasted	1 ounce	14
Catfish; breaded and fried	3 ounces	11
Caviar, red granular	1 tablespoon	3
Cereal, any variety	1 ounce	0–8
Cheese		
American	1 ounce	9
blue	1 ounce	8
brick	1 ounce	8
Brie	1 ounce	8
Camembert	1 ounce	7
caraway	1 ounce	8
cheddar	1 ounce	9
cheddar, reduced fat	1 ounce	2
Cheshire	1 ounce	9
Colby	1 ounce	9
Edam	1 ounce	8
feta	1 ounce	6
fondue	½ cup	18
fontina	1 ounce	9
gjetost	1 ounce	8
Gouda	1 ounce	8
Gruyère	1 ounce	9
Limburger	1 ounce	8
Monterey Jack	1 ounce	9
mozzarella	1 ounce	6
mozzarella, part skim	1 ounce	5
Muenster	1 ounce	9
Parmesan, grated	1 tablespoon	2

Food	Serving Size	Fat Grams
Parmesan	1 ounce	7
Port du Salut	1 ounce	8
provolone	1 ounce	8
ricotta, part skim	½ cup	10
ricotta, whole milk	½ cup	16
Romano	1 ounce	8
Roquefort	1 ounce	9
Swiss	1 ounce	8
Tilsit	1 ounce	7
Chicken		
a la king	¾ cup	16
back, meat only; stewed	1 ounce	3
boneless; breaded and fried	1 piece (.6 ounce)	3
boneless; breaded and fried	6 pieces (4.6 ounces)	18
boneless; breaded and fried, with barbecue sauce	6 pieces (4.6 ounces)	18
boneless; breaded and fried, with honey	6 pieces (4 ounces)	18
boneless; breaded and fried, with mustard sauce	6 pieces (4.6 ounces)	19
boneless; breaded and fried, with sweet-and-sour sauce	6 pieces (4.6 ounces)	18
breast, meat only; roasted	½ breast (3 ounces)	3
cacciatore	¾ cup	24
canned with broth	1 can (5 ounces)	11
chicken and dumplings	¾ cup	12
chicken and noodles	¾ cup	6
chicken roll, light meat	1 slice (1 ounce)	2
dark meat; breaded and fried	2 pieces (5.2 ounces)	27
drumstick, meat only; roasted	1.5 ounces	2
fillet sandwich	1	29
fillet sandwich with cheese	1	39

fricassee	¾ cup	17
light meat; breaded and fried	2 pieces (5.7 ounces)	30
neck, meat and skin; simmered	1 (1.3 ounces)	7
paprikash	¾ cup	5
skin only; roasted	from ½ chicken (2 ounces)	23
thigh, meat only; roasted	1 (1.8 ounces)	6
wing, meat and skin; roasted	1 (1.2 ounces)	7
Chili con carne	1 cup	8
Chitterlings, pork; simmered	3 ounces	24
Cisco; smoked	3 ounces	10
Clams		
breaded and fried	3 ounces	9
clam sauce, white	½ cup	22
cooked	3 ounces	2
raw	3 ounces	1
Cocoa, hot	1 cup	9
Coconut		
cream, canned	1 tablespoon	3
dried, toasted	1 ounce	13
milk, canned	1 tablespoon	3
raw	1 piece	15
Cod		
Atlantic; cooked	3 ounces	1
roe	3.5 ounces	2
Coffee Whiteners		
liquid, non-dairy	½ ounce	2
powder, non-dairy	1 teaspoon	tr
Coleslaw	¾ cup	11
Cookie		
animal crackers	1 box (2.3 ounces)	9
chocolate chip	1 (.4 ounce)	4
fig bar	1 (.5 ounce)	tr
fortune cookie	1 (.5 ounce)	4
gingersnap	1 (.25 ounce)	1
graham cracker	4	3
graham cracker, chocolate covered	2	6

The Fat Attack Plan FAT COUNTER (*cont.*)

Food	Serving Size	Fat Grams
lady finger	1	tr
lemon bar	1 (1 ounce)	5
macaroon	1 (.5 ounce)	2
molasses	1 (1.1 ounces)	5
oatmeal with raisin	1 (.5 ounce)	3
peanut butter	1 (.5 ounce)	3
sugar	1 (.4 ounce)	2
Corn		
chips	1 ounce	9
hush puppies	5	12
on the cob with butter	1 ear	3
Cottage Cheese		
1%	½ cup	1
2%	½ cup	2
creamed	½ cup	5
Crab		
Alaska king; cooked	3 ounces	1
baked	1 crab (2 ounces)	1
blue; cooked	3 ounces	2
cakes	1 cake (2.1 ounces)	5
canned	3 ounces	1
deviled	½ cup	12
imperial	½ cup	8
soft shell; fried	1 crab (4.4 ounces)	18
stew	½ cup	7
Crayfish; cooked	3 ounces	1
Cream		
half-and-half	1 tablespoon	2
heavy whipping	1 tablespoon	6
heavy; whipped	½ cup	22
light coffee	1 tablespoon	3
Cream Cheese		
Neufchâtel	1 ounce	7

regular	1 ounce	10
whipped	1 ounce	10

Croissant

plain	1	12
with egg and cheese	1	25
with egg, cheese, and bacon	1	28
with egg, cheese, and ham	1	34
with egg, cheese, and sausage	1	38

Custard

baked	½ cup	7
zabaglione	½ cup	7

Danish Pastry

cheese	1 (3 ounces)	25
fruit	1 (2.3 ounces)	13
fruit	1 (3 ounces)	16
plain	1 (2 ounces)	12
plain	1 (3 ounces)	17

Doughnut

cake type, plain	1 (1.5 ounces)	8
cake type, sugared	1 (1.6 ounces)	8
jelly	1 (2.3 ounces)	9
raised, plain	1 (1.5 ounces)	11

Duck, meat only; roasted	3.5 ounces	11
Eel; cooked	3 ounces	13

Egg

chicken	1	5
deviled	2 halves	13
duck	1	10
egg and cheese sandwich	1	19
egg foo yong	1 (5.1 ounces)	10
omelet, 2 eggs, butter, milk	1	14
salad	½ cup	28
sandwich with ham and cheese	1	16
scrambled	2 eggs	15
white only	1	tr
yolk only	1	5

Eggnog	1 cup	19

Food	Serving Size	Fat Grams
English Muffin		
with butter	1	6
with cheese and sausage	1	24
with egg, cheese, and Canadian bacon	1	20
with egg, cheese, and sausage	1	31
Fat		
lard	1 tablespoon	13
pork-back fat	1 ounce	25
shortening, vegetable	1 tablespoon	13
tallow (beef)	1 tablespoon	13
Filberts		
dry roasted	1 ounce	19
oil roasted	1 ounce	18
Fish (SEE ALSO INDIVIDUAL NAMES)		
fillet; battered	1 (3 ounces)	11
fillet; breaded	1 (3 ounces)	11
sandwich with tartar sauce	1	23
sandwich with tartar sauce and cheese	1	29
Flatfish; cooked	3 ounces	1
Flounder; cooked	3 ounces	1
French Toast		
french toast sticks	5 sticks	29
plain	1 slice	7
with butter	2 slices	19
Frogs' Legs; fried	1 (.8 ounce)	5
Gefilte Fish, sweet recipe	1 piece (1.5 ounces)	1
Goose, meat only; roasted	5 ounces	18
Gravy		
au jus	1 cup	tr
beef	1 cup	5
chicken	1 cup	14
mushroom	1 cup	6
turkey	1 cup	5

Grouper; cooked	3 ounces	1
Haddock		
cooked	3 ounces	1
roe	3.5 ounces	2
smoked	3 ounces	1
Halibut		
Atlantic; cooked	3 ounces	2
Pacific; cooked	3 ounces	2
Ham		
canned	3 ounces	13
canned, extra lean	3 ounces	7
croquettes	1 (3.1 ounces)	14
salad	½ cup	23
sandwich with cheese	1	15
sandwich with egg and cheese	1	16
sliced, extra lean	1 slice (1 ounce)	1
sliced, regular	1 slice (1 ounce)	3
steak, extra lean, boneless	3 ounces	3
whole, lean only; roasted	3 ounces	5
Hazelnuts		
dry roasted	1 ounce	19
oil roasted	1 ounce	18
Herring		
Atlantic; cooked	3 ounces	10
canned with tomato sauce	1.9 ounces	6
kippered, fillet	1.4 ounces	5
pickled	1 ounce	6
Hot Dogs		
beef	1 (1.5 ounces)	13
beef and pork	1 (1.75 ounces)	17
chicken	1 (1.5 ounces)	9
corn dog	1	19
pork and cheese	1 (1.5 ounces)	12
turkey	1 (1.5 ounces)	8
with bun	1	14
with bun and chili	1	13
Hummus	⅓ cup	7
Ice Cream		
orange sherbet	½ cup	2

Food	Serving Size	Fat Grams
sundae, caramel	1 small (5.4 ounces)	9
sundae, hot fudge	1 small (5.4 ounces)	9
sundae, strawberry	1 small (5.4 ounces)	8
vanilla ice cream (10% fat)	½ cup	7
vanilla ice cream (16% fat)	½ cup	12
vanilla ice milk	½ cup	3
vanilla, soft serve	½ cup	12
Lamb		
curry	¾ cup	17
leg, without bone, lean only; roasted	3 ounces	6
loin chop, with bone, lean and fat; broiled	1 (2.5 ounces)	21
patty, lean and fat; cooked	3 ounces	16
rib chop, with bone, lean and fat; cooked	1 (2.4 ounces)	24
shank, lean and fat; cooked	3.2 ounces	25
shoulder, without bone, lean only; roasted	3 ounces	9
stew	¾ cup	5
Liver		
beef; pan fried	3 ounces	7
chicken; cooked	1 (.6 ounce)	1
pork; braised	3 ounces	4
Lobster		
cooked	3 ounces	1
Newburg	1 cup	27
Luncheon Meats/Cold Cuts		
barbecue loaf, beef	1 slice (23 grams)	2
beerwurst	1 slice (23 grams)	7
bologna, beef	1 slice (23 grams)	7
bologna, beef and pork	1 slice (23 grams)	7
bologna, pork	1 slice (23 grams)	5

braunschweiger	1 ounce	9
dried beef	1 ounce	1
Dutch brand loaf, pork and beef	1 slice (28 grams)	5
ham & cheese loaf	1 slice (28 grams)	11
headcheese, pork	1 slice (28 grams)	4
honey loaf, pork and beef	1 slice (28 grams)	1
liverwurst	1 ounce	8
luxury loaf, pork	1 slice (28 grams)	5
mortadella, beef and pork	1 slice (15 grams)	4
olive loaf, pork	1 slice (28 grams)	5
pastrami	1 slice (28 grams)	8
peppered loaf, pork and beef	1 slice (28 grams)	2
pickle and pimiento loaf, pork	1 slice (28 grams)	6
salami, cooked, beef	1 slice (23 grams)	5
salami, hard, pork	1 slice (10 grams)	4
submarine sandwich with ham, salami, cheese, lettuce, tomato, onion, and oil	1	19
Macadamia Nuts		
dried	1 ounce	21
oil roasted	1 ounce	22
Mackerel		
Atlantic; cooked	3 ounces	15
Spanish; cooked	3 ounces	5
Margarine		
reduced-calorie corn oil	1 teaspoon	2
regular corn oil	1 teaspoon	4
soft corn oil	1 teaspoon	4
Mayonnaise		
mayonnaise-type salad dressing	1 tablespoon	5
reduced calorie	1 tablespoon	3
regular	1 tablespoon	11
Mexican Food		
burrito with apples	1 small (2.6 ounces)	10
burrito with apples	1 large (5.4 ounces)	20
burrito with beans	2 (7.6 ounces)	14
burrito with beans and cheese	2 (6.5 ounces)	12

The Fat Attack Plan FAT COUNTER (*cont.*)

Food	Serving Size	Fat Grams
burrito with beans and chili peppers	2 (7.2 ounces)	15
burrito with beans and meat	2 (8.1 ounces)	18
burrito with beans, cheese, and beef	2 (7.1 ounces)	13
burrito with beans, cheese, and chili peppers	2 (11.8 ounces)	23
burrito with beef	2 (7.7 ounces)	21
burrito with beef and chili peppers	2 (7.1 ounces)	17
burrito with beef, cheese, and chili peppers	2 (10.7 ounces)	25
burrito with cherries	1 small (2.6 ounces)	10
burrito with cherries	1 large (5.4 ounces)	20
chimichanga with beef	1 (6.1 ounces)	20
chimichanga with beef and cheese	1 (6.4 ounces)	23
chimichanga with beef and red chili peppers	1 (6.7 ounces)	19
chimichanga with beef, cheese, and red chili peppers	1 (6.3 ounces)	18
enchilada, eggplant	1	5
enchilada with cheese	1 (5.7 ounces)	19
enchilada with cheese and beef	1 (6.7 ounces)	18
enchirito with cheese, beef, and beans	1 (6.8 ounces)	16
frijoles with cheese	1 cup (5.9 ounces)	8
nachos with cheese	6 to 8 nachos (4 ounces)	19
nachos with cheese and jalapeño peppers	6 to 8 nachos (7.2 ounces)	34
nachos with cheese, beans, ground beef, and peppers	6 to 8 nachos (8.9 ounces)	31
nachos with cinnamon and sugar	6 to 8 nachos (3.8 ounces)	36
taco	1 small (6 ounces)	21
taco	1 large (9.2 ounces)	32

taco salad	1½ cups	15
taco salad with chili con carne	1½ cups	13
tamale	1 (3.9 ounces)	8
tortilla; baked or steamed	1 (.7 ounce)	tr
tostada with beans and cheese	1 (5.1 ounces)	10
tostada with beans, beef, and cheese	1 (7.9 ounces)	17
tostada with beef and cheese	1 (5.7 ounces)	16
tostada with guacamole	1 (4.6 ounces)	23

Milk

1%	1 cup	3
2%	1 cup	5
buttermilk	1 cup	2
chocolate, low fat, 1%	1 cup	3
chocolate, low fat, 2%	1 cup	5
chocolate, whole	1 cup	8
condensed, sweetened	1 ounce	3
evaporated	1 ounce	2
evaporated, skim	1 ounce	tr
nonfat dry	¼ cup	tr
skim	1 cup	tr
skim, protein fortified	1 cup	1
whole	1 cup	8

Milkshake

chocolate	10 ounces	11
strawberry	10 ounces	8
vanilla	10 ounces	8

Muffin

apple	1 (1.6 ounces)	7
blueberry	1 (1.6 ounces)	7
bran	1 (1.9 ounces)	4
corn	1 (1.6 ounces)	9
orange	1 (1.6 ounces)	6
plain	1 (1.6 ounces)	8
whole wheat	1 (1.6 ounces)	3

Mullet; cooked	3 ounces	4

Mussel

cooked	3 ounces	4
raw	3 ounces	2

The Fat Attack Plan FAT COUNTER (*cont.*)

Food	Serving Size	Fat Grams
Noodles		
egg	½ cup	1
noodle pudding	½ cup	7
Oil		
almond	1 tablespoon	14
canola	1 tablespoon	14
coconut	1 tablespoon	14
corn	1 tablespoon	14
cottonseed	1 tablespoon	14
hazelnut	1 tablespoon	14
olive	1 tablespoon	14
peanut	1 tablespoon	14
safflower	1 tablespoon	14
sesame	1 tablespoon	14
soybean	1 tablespoon	14
sunflower	1 tablespoon	14
walnut	1 tablespoon	14
wheat germ	1 tablespoon	14
Olives		
green	4 medium	2
ripe	2 large	2
Onion Rings; breaded and fried	8 to 9 rings (2.9 ounces)	16
Oriental Food		
chicken teriyaki	¾ cup	27
chop suey with meat	1 cup	7
chow mein noodles	½ cup	5
chow mein with chicken	1 cup	10
wonton; fried	½ cup	8
Oyster		
eastern; breaded and fried	3 ounces	11
eastern, canned	3 ounces	2
eastern; cooked	3 ounces	4
eastern, raw	6 medium	2
Pacific, raw	6 medium	6

Rockefeller	3 oysters	2
stew	1 cup	18

Pancakes

buckwheat	1 (6″ diameter)	3
buttermilk	1 (6″ diameter)	5
plain	1 (6″ diameter)	5
potato	1 (4″ diameter)	6
with butter and syrup	3 pancakes	14
zucchini	1 (4″ diameter)	3

Pasta Dinners

lasagna	2½″ × 2½″ (8.8 ounces)	21
macaroni and cheese	¾ cup	17
manicotti	¾ cup	12
rigatoni with sausage sauce	¾ cup	12
spaghetti with meatballs and tomato sauce	1 cup	12
spaghetti with tomato sauce and cheese	1 cup	2

Pâté

chicken liver	1 ounce	4
goose liver, smoked	1 ounce	12
liver	1 ounce	8

Peanuts

peanut butter, chunk style	1 tablespoon	8
peanut butter, smooth style	1 tablespoon	8
dry roasted	1 ounce	14
oil roasted	1 ounce	14

Pecans

dry roasted	1 ounce	18
oil roasted	1 ounce	20

Perch; Atlantic; cooked	3 ounces	2

Pie

apple	⅐ of 9″ pie	19
banana cream	⅐ of 9″ pie	16
blackberry	⅐ of 9″ pie	15
blueberry	⅐ of 9″ pie	19
butterscotch	⅐ of 9″ pie	21

The Fat Attack Plan FAT COUNTER (*cont.*)

Food	Serving Size	Fat Grams
cherry	⅐ of 9" pie	20
chess	⅐ of 9" pie	42
chocolate	⅐ of 9" pie	19
chocolate meringue	⅐ of 9" pie	19
coconut custard	⅐ of 9" pie	18
crust only	⅐ of 9" pie	9
custard	⅐ of 9" pie	18
grasshopper	⅐ of 9" pie	20
key lime	⅐ of 9" pie	16
lemon chiffon	⅐ of 9" pie	21
lemon meringue	⅐ of 9" pie	16
mince	⅐ of 9" pie	21
peach	⅐ of 9" pie	20
pecan	⅐ of 9" pie	33
pineapple chiffon	⅐ of 9" pie	18
pumpkin	⅐ of 9" pie	15
raisin	⅐ of 9" pie	27
rhubarb	⅐ of 9" pie	19
snack pie, apple	1 (2.5 ounces)	14
snack pie, cherry	1 (2.5 ounces)	14
snack pie, lemon	1 (2.5 ounces)	14
squash	⅐ of 9" pie	17
strawberry	⅐ of 9" pie	12
Pierogi	¾ cup	19
Pigs' Ears and Feet		
ear; simmered	1 (3.7 ounces)	12
feet, pickled	1 ounce	5
feet; simmered	2.5 ounces	9
Pike, northern; cooked	3 ounces	1
Pine Nuts		
pignolia, dried	1 ounce	14
piñon, dried	1 ounce	17
Pistachios, dry roasted	1 ounce	15
Pizza		
cheese	⅐ of 10" pie	4

cheese	⅛ of 12" pie	3
cheese and pepperoni	⅛ of 12" pie	5
cheese and sausage	⅛ of 14" pie	16
cheese, meat, and vegetables	⅛ of 12" pie	4
Pollack; cooked	3 ounces	1

Popcorn
air popped	1 cup	tr
popped with vegetable oil	1 cup	3
Popover	1 (1.4 ounces)	4

Pork
center loin, lean only; roasted	3 ounces	11
center loin chop, lean and fat; broiled	1 chop (3.1 ounces)	19
loin, lean only; roasted	3 ounces	12
loin blade chop, lean and fat; broiled	1 chop (3.1 ounces)	27
loin center rib chop, lean and fat; broiled	1 chop (2.7 ounces)	23
rib chop, lean and fat; broiled	1 chop (2.6 ounces)	20
salt pork	1 ounce	23
shoulder, lean only; roasted	3 ounces	11
sirloin chop, lean and fat; broiled	1 chop (2.8 ounces)	21
spareribs, lean and fat; braised	3 ounces	26
tenderloin, lean only; roasted	3 ounces	4

Pot Pie
beef	4¼" diameter	33
chicken	11 ounces	46
turkey	10.6 ounces	47

Potatoes
au gratin	½ cup	9
au gratin with cheese	½ cup	10
baked	1	tr
baked with cheese sauce	1	29
baked with cheese sauce and bacon	1	26
baked with cheese sauce and broccoli	1	21
baked with cheese sauce and chili	1	22

Food	Serving Size	Fat Grams
baked with sour cream and chives	1	22
french fries	10 strips	4
french fries	1 regular order (2.7 ounces)	12
french fries	1 large order (4 ounces)	19
hash browns	½ cup	9
mashed	½ cup	4
O'Brien	1 cup	3
potato chips	10 chips	7
potato chips	1 ounce	10
potato puffs	½ cup	7
salad	½ cup	10
scalloped	½ cup	5
Pudding		
bread with raisins	½ cup	5
chocolate	½ cup	4
corn	½ cup	1
pumpkin	½ cup	5
rice with raisins	½ cup	6
tapioca	½ cup	6
vanilla	½ cup	4
Pumpkin Seeds; dried	1 ounce	13
Quiche, lorraine	⅙ of 9″ pie	27
Rabbit; stewed	3.5 ounces	10
Rockfish; cooked	3 ounces	2
Sablefish; smoked	3 ounces	17
Salad		
chef without dressing with turkey, ham, and cheese	1½ cups	16
tossed without dressing	1½ cups	tr
tossed without dressing with cheese and egg	1½ cups	6
tossed without dressing with chicken	1½ cups	2

tossed without dressing with pasta and seafood	1½ cups	21
tossed without dressing with shrimp	1½ cups	2
Salad Dressing		
blue cheese	1 tablespoon	8
French	1 tablespoon	6
French, reduced calorie	1 tablespoon	1
Italian	1 tablespoon	7
Italian, reduced calorie	1 tablespoon	2
Russian	1 tablespoon	8
Russian, reduced calorie	1 tablespoon	1
sesame seed	1 tablespoon	7
Thousand Island	1 tablespoon	6
Thousand Island, reduced calorie	1 tablespoon	2
vinegar and oil	1 tablespoon	8
Salmon		
chum with bone, canned	3 ounces	5
coho; cooked	3 ounces	6
pink with bone, canned	3 ounces	5
salmon cake	3.4 ounces	15
salmon rice loaf	½" slice	16
smoked, chinook	3 ounces	4
sockeye; cooked	3 ounces	9
sockeye with bone, canned	3 ounces	6
Sardine		
Atlantic, in oil with bone	2 ounces	3
Pacific, in brine and mustard	1 large (.7 ounce)	2
Pacific with tomato sauce with bone	1 ounce	5
Sauce		
barbecue	¼ cup	1
béarnaise	¼ cup	17
cheese	¼ cup	4
curry	¼ cup	4
hollandaise with butter	¼ cup	5
mushroom	½ cup	5
sour cream	¼ cup	8
sweet and sour	¼ cup	tr
teriyaki	¼ cup	tr
white	¼ cup	3

The Fat Attack Plan FAT COUNTER (*cont.*)

Food	Serving Size	Fat Grams
Sausage		
bratwurst, pork; cooked	1 ounce	7
country style, pork; cooked	1 ounce	8
Italian, pork; cooked	1 link (2 ounces)	17
kielbasa	1 ounce	8
knockwurst, pork and beef	1 ounce	8
pork and beef; cooked	1 ounce	10
pork; cooked	1 ounce	8
smoked, beef	1 (1.4 ounces)	12
smoked, pork	1 ounce	10
smoked, pork and beef	1 ounce	10
Vienna, canned, beef and pork	1 ounce	4
Scallop; breaded and fried	1 large	3
Scone	1 (1.4 ounce)	6
Sesame		
butter	1 tablespoon	8
seeds, roasted and toasted	1 tablespoon	14
tahini	1 tablespoon	8
Sheepshead Fish; cooked	3 ounces	4
Shellfish Substitute		
crab, imitation	3 ounces	1
scallop, imitation	3 ounces	1
surimi	3 ounces	1
Shrimp		
breaded and fried	3 ounces	10
canned	3 ounces	2
fresh; cooked	3 ounces	1
jambalaya	¾ cup	5
stew	1 cup	14
Smelt, rainbow; cooked	3 ounces	3
Snail; cooked	3 ounces	1
Snapper; cooked	3 ounces	1
Sole; cooked	3 ounces	1

Soufflé

cheese	1 cup	25
grand marnier	1 cup	4
lemon, chilled	1 cup	tr
raspberry, chilled	1 cup	tr
spinach	1 cup	18

Soup

asparagus, cream of	1 cup	8
bean with bacon	1 cup	6
bean with frankfurters	1 cup	7
beef broth	1 cup	1
beef noodle	1 cup	3
black bean	1 cup	2
black bean turtle	1 cup	tr
celery, cream of	1 cup	10
cheese	1 cup	15
chicken broth	1 cup	1
chicken, cream of	1 cup	11
chicken gumbo	1 cup	1
chicken noodle	1 cup	2
chicken rice	1 cup	2
chicken vegetable	1 cup	3
clam chowder, Manhattan	1 cup	2
clam chowder, New England	1 cup	7
consommé	1 cup	0
corn and cheese chowder	1 cup	15
corn chowder	1 cup	11
escarole	1 cup	2
gazpacho	1 cup	tr
Greek	1 cup	2
hot and sour	1 cup	2
leek	1 cup	2
lentil	1 cup	2
lentil with ham	1 cup	3
minestrone	1 cup	3
mock turtle	1 cup	14
mushroom, cream of	1 cup	14
mushroom with beef stock	1 cup	4
onion	1 cup	2
oxtail	1 cup	3

Food	Serving Size	Fat Grams
pea	1 cup	3
pepperpot	1 cup	5
potato, cream of	1 cup	6
Scotch broth	1 cup	3
seafood chowder	1 cup	6
shrimp, cream of	1 cup	9
split pea with ham	1 cup	4
tomato	1 cup	2
tomato bisque	1 cup	7
tomato rice	1 cup	3
turkey vegetable	1 cup	3
vegetable	1 cup	tr
vegetable with beef broth	1 cup	2
vichyssoise	1 cup	6
wonton	1 cup	3
Sour Cream		
imitation	1 tablespoon	3
regular	1 tablespoon	3
Soy		
lecithin	1 tablespoon	14
soy milk	1 cup	5
soybeans, dry roasted	½ cup	19
Spaghetti Sauce		
marinara	1 cup	8
regular	1 cup	10
Squid; fried	3 ounces	6
Stuffing		
bread; made with fat	½ cup	15
bread; made with egg and fat	½ cup	7
sausage	½ cup	11
Sturgeon		
cooked	3 ounces	4
smoked	3 ounces	4
Sunflower Seeds		
dry roasted	1 ounce	14

oil roasted	1 ounce	16
sunflower butter	1 tablespoon	8
Swordfish; cooked	3 ounces	4
Tofu		
regular	4 ounces	6
fried	1 ounce	6
Tongue		
beef; simmered	3 ounces	18
pork; simmered	3 ounces	16
Trout, rainbow; cooked	3 ounces	4
Tuna		
bluefin; cooked	3 ounces	5
light, canned in oil	3 ounces	7
light, canned in water	3 ounces	tr
submarine sandwich with lettuce and oil	1	28
tuna salad	½ cup	8
white, canned in oil	3 ounces	7
white, canned in water	3 ounces	2
Turkey		
bologna	1 slice (1 ounce)	4
breast	1 ounce	tr
canned with broth	2.5 ounces	5
dark meat without skin; roasted	3 ounces	6
ham	1 slice (1 ounce)	3
light meat without skin; roasted	4 ounces	3
loaf	2 slices (1.5 ounces)	1
neck meat; simmered	1 neck (5.3 ounces)	11
pastrami	1 slice (1 ounce)	4
roll	1 slice (1 ounce)	2
salami	1 slice (1 ounce)	4
stew	¾ cup	9
sticks, breaded, battered; fried	1 stick (2.3 ounces)	11
wing, meat and skin; roasted	1 wing (8.3 ounces)	27

Food	Serving Size	Fat Grams
Veal		
cutlet; braised	3 ounces	9
loin chop, lean and fat; cooked	1 chop (3.9 ounces)	11
loin roast, with bone, lean and fat; roasted	3 ounces	11
parmigiana	4.2 ounces	18
rib chop with bone, lean and fat; cooked	1 chop (3.5 ounces)	17
round, patty; cooked	3 ounces	9
shoulder, without bone, lean only; braised	3 ounces	5
veal loaf	1 slice (4.7 ounces)	17
Yogurt, any flavor	6–8 ounces	0–10
Walnuts		
black, dried	1 ounce	16
English, dried	1 ounce	18
Whipped Topping		
cream, pressurized	1 tablespoon	1
non-dairy, frozen	1 tablespoon	1
non-dairy, pressurized	1 tablespoon	1
Whiting; cooked	3 ounces	1

10 *In Control at the Supermarket*

HOW TO SHOP WHEN YOU'RE ATTACKING YOUR FAT

Navigating through the maze of choices in a typical supermarket can be a dieter's nightmare. Obstacles and temptations are *everywhere:* end-of-aisle displays hawking bargains, food tastings for new products, clever labels that promise everlasting health with words like "lite," "high-fiber," "low-cholesterol," and "low-fat." If you're committed to good health, going up and down the supermarket aisles is a little like treading through a minefield. All your good intentions can be blown to pieces by the time you reach the check-out counter.

With the help of the Fat Attack Target and some supermarket savvy, you *can* get through this jungle of temptations. But you have to make a plan of attack.

Shop the perimeter of the store first—the aisles on the far left and right and across the back. In most stores, these aisles contain fresh fruits and vegetables, meat, poultry, fish, dairy products, and breads. These are the basic, nutritious foods you're planning your meals around. Many are free (the center of the Fat Attack Target). Others are in the middle, "some fat" ring of the Target (foods to choose most often). By the time you've shopped the outer aisles, your basket should be pretty full. Now go up and down the inner aisles, picking up the few extra items you need.

But beware of land mines! End-of-aisle displays are meant to grab your attention, enticing you to buy a new product or a weekly special. Keep in mind that it's not a bargain if you don't need it. Cents-off coupons, even double-value ones, are only worthwhile if they're for products that fit into your eating plan. We're not saying you can never buy a cookie or a doughnut again. But plan these purchases; make a decision to fit these choices into your eating plan *before* you go shopping. Don't make a spontaneous, and possibly wrong, decision at the store.

Learning from Labels

You don't have to have a degree in nutrition to read a nutrition label, but it sure helps. The standard nutrition label is full of valuable information, and if legislators are successful, even more will be on it in the near future.

It's fine if you want to take the time and effort to read the entire label. You certainly can't make informed decisions at the market *without* looking at labels, no matter what aisle you're in. But to stay In Control you have to look at only one or the other of two things to determine if the food is a good choice: the number of grams of fat in the food, if the label tells you that, or the list of ingredients the food contains.

First, check the grams of fat in one serving. You're looking for foods that are low in fat. That means *a food should have no more than three grams of fat per one hundred calories to fit into your Fat Attack Plan*. Following are two examples of ready-to-heat entrées. The labels tell you that the first food is a good choice but the second one is not.

A LOW-FAT CHOICE

NUTRITION INFORMATION PER SERVING

Servings per container	2
Serving size	1 cup
Calories	160
Protein	5 grams
Carbohydrate	31 grams
Fat	1 gram

This ready-to-heat main dish has less than one gram of fat per one hundred calories, far below the suggested three grams per one hundred calories. It's a good low-fat choice.

A HIGH-FAT CHOICE:

NUTRITION INFORMATION PER SERVING

Servings per container	4
Serving size	1 cup
Calories	170
Protein	6 grams
Carbohydrate	18 grams
Fat	8 grams

This ready-to-heat main dish has more than three grams of fat per one hundred calories. Leave this high-fat choice on the supermarket shelf!

If there isn't a nutrition label, look at the list of ingredients. Every packaged food (except for a few items like mayonnaise, ketchup, and ice cream, all of which have standard ingredients) must include an ingredients list. Ingredients are listed by weight, from most to least. You can tell at a glance that a choice is high in fat if a fatty ingredient is one of the first on the list.

Below are two examples of ingredients lists from cookie packages. The first is a low-fat choice, the second is not.

A LOW-FAT CHOICE:

INGREDIENTS: Enriched flour, whole-wheat flour, sugar, molasses, soybean oil, honey, baking soda, cinnamon, baking powder, salt.

These cookies have one source of fat, soybean oil, and it is halfway down the list. You can assume that these cookies are not very high in fat.

A HIGH-FAT CHOICE:

INGREDIENTS: Cocoa butter, wheat flour, hydrogenated coconut oil, hydrogenated peanut oil, sugar, cocoa, whole milk, hazelnuts, egg yolk, baking powder, spice, vanillin (an artificial flavor).

These cookies have six sources of fat, so it's a good bet they *are* high in fat. You can easily identify sources of fat because they're the foods in the outer rings of the Fat Attack Target. If some terms for fat are unfamiliar to you, the list below should be helpful.

INGREDIENTS HIGH IN FAT

Animal fat	Mayonnaise
Beef suet	Nuts
Butter	Palm-kernel oil
Cheese	Palm oil
Cocoa butter	Partially hydrogenated oil,
Coconut	any kind
Coconut oil	Seeds
Cream	Shortening
Egg yolk	Sour cream
Hydrogenated oil,	Vegetable oil
any kind	Vegetable shortening
Lard	Whole egg
Liquid oil, any kind	Whole milk
Margarine	Whole-milk solids

Remember, if you want to avoid fat, don't buy foods that list fat as the first or second ingredient! And limit foods that list many fats and oils as ingredients or that list fat as a main ingredient.

Smart Shopping

Now that you know what to look out for and how to see past the disguises that fat can wear, let's put your new knowledge to work.

FRUITS AND VEGETABLES

Load up your shopping cart with these. Low in fat, high in fiber, and rich in nutrients, these foods are near the center of the Fat Attack Target. Use a wide variety, in unlimited amounts. But pass up the olives, coconuts, and avocados—all high in fat—unless you've worked them into your fat allowance ahead of time.

BREAD, CEREAL, PASTA, BEANS, RICE, AND OTHER GRAINS

This is another group of foods at the center of the Fat Attack Target. Buy ample amounts and use them freely at each meal or snack. Choose whole-grain varieties for a fiber bonus; avoid granola cereals and specialty breads, like nut bread or banana bread, which are higher in fat.

MEAT

You don't need to stop eating red meat just because you're eating less fat. Just select lean, well-trimmed cuts and keep the portion sizes moderate—three to four ounces per person. It's important to know that meats graded "Select" have less fat than "Choice" or "Prime" cuts. Some producers are even marketing meat with less trimmable fat (fat surrounding the meat) and less marbling (fat in the muscle of the meat). As time goes on, more genetically bred low-fat meat will probably be available.

LEAN CUTS OF MEAT

Beef	*Veal*	*Pork*	*Lamb*
Round	All trimmed cuts	Tenderloin	Leg
Sirloin	(except ground)	Leg (fresh)	Arm
Chuck		Shoulder	Loin
Loin		(arm or picnic)	

Most processed meat, such as bologna, salami, and hot dogs, are very high in fat. Try not to use these more than once in a while. The same goes for spare ribs and bacon.

Organ meats, like liver and kidneys, are relatively low in fat but unusually high in cholesterol, so don't buy them often. Once or twice a month is fine.

POULTRY

Chicken, turkey, and cornish hen are your best choices. But cook and eat them *without* the skin. Ground turkey, lower in fat than ground beef, pork, or veal, makes a great substitute for any of those fattier meats. Duck and goose, and poultry products like turkey bologna and chicken hot dogs, are much higher in fat than plain chicken or turkey. Once in a while they're fine, but don't buy them regularly.

FISH AND SHELLFISH

Most fish is lower in fat than meat is. If you buy frozen varieties, stick to plain choices, minus the butter, cream sauce, or breading. Those with tomato sauce are probably fine; check the label. If you're buying canned fish, choose the varieties packed in water or broth rather than in oil. If you like sardines, choose those packed in mustard or tomato sauce instead of in oil.

MILK AND YOGURT

Skim milk and 1% milk are the best choices. If you're finding it hard to switch to a low-fat milk, ease into the choice. Try 2% milk rather than whole milk for a few weeks, then switch to 1% and finally to skim. If you like the creaminess of whole milk, try drinking buttermilk, which is actually a skim-milk product. Buttermilk cultures, not fat, are what make it thick.

Non-dairy creamers (also known as coffee whiteners) have as much fat as half-and-half. And many brands use tropical oils—palm, palm-kernel, and coconut oils—which are high in cholesterol-raising saturated fat. If you find it hard to give up the cream in your coffee, try whole milk. Once you've made the change to a low-fat milk for regular use, you'll be amazed how "creamy" whole milk tastes. Indulging yourself with a little in your coffee or tea will be very satisfying.

Low- and nonfat yogurts are good milk substitutes, and they provide all the nutrients in milk, without the fat. Buy flavors that have less than two grams of fat in a one-cup serving.

CHEESE

The amount of meat we eat each year is going down, but the amount of cheese we eat is going up! That's because many people still make a common mistake: When they cut down on meat they think it's okay to eat more cheese. Regular cheese is *very* high in fat. In fact, you can think of it the way you think of butter: It's almost all fat. Try low-fat varieties and use very small amounts of the regular kind. Grating makes a little go a long way. Aged, very hard cheeses, like locatelli and sapsago are lower in fat, and using small amounts can add a good punch of flavor.

Check the labels of new "light" or "low-fat" cheeses. If they contain five grams of fat or less per ounce, they qualify as good choices.

If you like cream cheese, you can save yourself some fat in a couple of ways. By weight, both whipped cream cheese and regular cream cheese have ten grams of fat per ounce. But whipped cream cheese is fluffier, so a little goes further; there are three tablespoons in one ounce, compared with two tablespoons per ounce for regular cream cheese. Then there's also reduced-fat (light) cream cheese; it has only half as much fat as the regular kind.

EGGS

Whenever they're available, buy medium or small eggs, because they have less cholesterol; eat no more than three or four a week. Eggs have five grams of fat apiece and it's all in the yolk (all the cholesterol is there, too), so discard the yolks and use only the whites as often as possible. Don't be fooled by egg substitutes; not all of them are low in fat. Some replace part of the egg fat with vegetable oil, resulting in a choice that's low in cholesterol but not low in fat. Read the label before you buy!

FATS AND OILS

Solid fats—butter, margarine, lard, and shortening—are higher in saturated fats than are liquid oils. Oils contain a lot of polyunsaturated and monounsaturated fats. Olive, canola, and soybean oils are the best choices because they're rich in "polys" and "monos" and are low in saturated fats. Don't be misled by "light" oils: They're not lower in fat, only lighter in color or flavor. **There are no low-fat oils on the market.** Don't be fooled.

Using cooking sprays can cut down on the amount of regular fat or oil you use—but spray lightly. Remember, these are still oil, and if you spray too long or too often you may wind up with too much fat.

Whipped butter and margarine have less fat per tablespoon than the stick variety because some air has been beaten in. "Diet" varieties have even less; these are made with added water, which allows them to spread further, so you use less. They're a good choice.

Light or "diet" mayonnaise often has half the fat of regular, but even so, it contains a lot. Mayonnaise-type salad dressings also have less fat than regular mayonnaise.

If you buy regular bottled salad dressings, use them sparingly. Low-fat or no-fat dressings are much better choices. Read the labels on "light" salad-dressing bottles to be sure they're actually lower in oil.

Sour cream is lower in fat than butter or mayonnaise, but it shouldn't be a regular choice. Don't be fooled by "imitation sour cream"; often the butterfat is taken out and an oil put in. You're just trading one fat for another, not lowering the total amount.

Just remember that no matter what fats you buy, you're better off using small amounts and working them into your daily menus with care. If you don't plan ahead, they can "eat up" your fat grams quickly.

FROZEN FOODS

In this aisle you need to rely on your shopping skills. Read the labels and check the ingredients lists. A good rule of thumb: the plainer the food, the lower in fat. Sauces, butter, batter, and breading all add fat.

Ice milk, sherbet, frozen yogurt, and frozen pudding are lower in fat than ice cream. Regular ice cream is lower in fat than "premium" or "gourmet" varieties. But sorbets, fruit ices, and frozen juice bars (without added cream) are virtually fat free and therefore make wonderful treats.

Frozen pies, cakes, pastries, and cookies can be very high in fat. Buy these only occasionally and keep your portions small. If you check the suggested serving size on the label, you'll see that it's often very small. This is how the producer fools you into thinking it's not such a bad choice. Don't fall for this labeling gimmick!

You can enjoy these sweets once in a while, though: Buy single-serving sizes of any of these frozen desserts and eat just one. That way, no matter what you pick, it will be hard to overdo it. And you can adjust your total fat intake for the day to allow a treat like this occasionally.

BAKERY ITEMS

Cakes, cookies, pies, croissants, muffins, biscuits, butter rolls, and dough-nuts are all reservoirs of fat. Before you eat one, place it on a paper napkin for a minute. If it leaves a greasy ring it's better left on the supermarket shelf the next time you shop. Eating any of these occasionally is fine, but the best of them still has more fat than "free foods" like regular bread and rolls.

When these choices aren't prepackaged and labeled it's hard to guess how much fat they have in them. But remember that a cookie that "snaps" when you break it is much lower in fat than one that bends. Good examples are gingersnaps and graham crackers. Fruit bars are also good. And there is one cake you can enjoy often—angel food cake. Its name hints at what a good choice it is; in fact, a slice is fat free.

CANDY, CHIPS, AND SNACKS

You can find just about everything in this aisle: high-fat choices, low-fat choices, and no-fat choices.

Potato chips, cheese puffs, tortilla chips, corn chips, buttered popcorn, and cheese-flavored popcorn may all be delicious, but they're all high in fat. An ounce of potato chips—that's ten chips—has more fat than two and a half teaspoons of butter! And how often do you eat just one ounce?

Most microwave popcorn is high in fat. Make your own popcorn by air-popping the kernels instead; prepared that way, it has only a trace of fat. So do pretzels.

Peanuts and other nuts can be pressed to make oil, so it stands to reason that they're high in fat. The same goes for seeds. A handful once in a while is fine, but if you eat them more often you'll be eating lots of "invisible" fat.

Almost everybody loves chocolate, but one of the main ingredients in chocolate is cocoa butter. When you see those words, think "fat!" In fact, think about chocolate as being equal in fat to cream cheese. Who wouldn't think twice before sitting down to eat a package of cream cheese?

One low-fat chocolate treat you can enjoy is snack-size, chocolate-covered peppermint patties. One of these has only one gram of fat. Marshmallows, hard candies, gumdrops, jelly beans, and licorice are all virtually fat free.

AT THE DELI COUNTER

The National Restaurant Association reports that on any day, twenty million people eat take-out food. Take-out cold meats, salads, and reheatable entrées are all available in most supermarkets today. But the amount of fat in these choices can vary almost as much as the selections available.

Sliced roast beef, turkey, and lean ham are the meat choices lowest in fat. For other cold cuts, select those marked "95% fat free." Salads with vinegar dressing are lower in fat than those made with mayonnaise or marinated in oil. Many delis are now making salads with "light" dressing or completely "undressed." These are options to try and see how fatty they really are. As you become more accustomed to a lower-fat diet, you'll get better at knowing a high-fat food just by the way it feels in your mouth.

Vinegar-dressed pasta or bean dishes—without lots of oil—are good entrées to take out. Barbecued chicken is good, too. Go easy on ribs, fried chicken, batter-dipped vegetables, pâté, and casseroles with cheese or cream sauce.

Check It Out

You've been up and down all the aisles and you're ready to head for the shortest check-out line. This is your last chance to change your mind! Before you start emptying your cart or basket, take one last look at what you've selected. If you have second thoughts about buying anything with a lot of fat in it, leave it behind.

Once you're home, empty your grocery bags and admire all your sensible purchases the way you would a new article of clothing. Remember, you "wear" what you buy at the supermarket, too!

11 *In Control in Your Kitchen*
TIPS FOR LOW-FAT COOKING

Funny, isn't it, that the center of activity in so many homes is the kitchen. It's where you chat over a meal or coffee with family or friends, where someone is almost always on the phone, where you sit to read the mail, where homework is often spread out right in the middle of everything else. Even at a party, they say, the *real* party is in the kitchen. Invariably, the kitchen is the center of the household.

In just the same way, your kitchen will be the control center for your Fat Attack Plan. Once you've done the marketing, chosen the right foods, and planned your meals, it's time to prepare the food and start cooking. There's no need to wonder what's in the things you eat when you make them yourself. Remember, *you* are In Control!

Just think of your kitchen, stocked with all the right foods, as your ally in your attack on fat. If you love to cook, then you're in your element. Coming up with new low-fat dishes and modifying the old ones will be a creative adventure. If you hate to cook, well, maybe you'll learn to like it better when you see what good-tasting, healthy foods you can prepare. And if you *really* hate to cook, start relying even more on your microwave. It's one of the best ways we know of to cook without added fat.

Planning Your Meals

Put your Fat Attack Target on the refrigerator or on the kitchen bulletin board; each meal you plan should feature ample amounts of the foods near the center of the Target. For example, if you're planning to make spaghetti and meatballs, cook lots of pasta, serve it with whole-wheat Italian bread, and make a big salad. But go easy on the meatballs; one or two are more than enough for a serving.

For a stir-fried dinner, heap on the vegetables and cook lots of rice, but cut back on the meat, fish, or poultry. Use the protein-rich food to top off the stir-fry, not to smother it. Or make a big pot of soup or stew featuring lots of vegetables, a little meat, seasonings, and lots of barley or rice. The best part of this kind of meal planning is that the portion sizes of those foods near the center of the Target—breads, rice, potatoes, cereal, pasta, beans, fruits, and vegetables—are unlimited.

Make a Little Change Here and There

Simple changes in cooking can significantly reduce the fat without sacrificing the flavor. Roast, steam, poach, bake, broil, grill, and microwave instead of frying or sautéing in butter or oil. When you do fry or sauté, stir-fry quickly in a nonstick pan, using cooking spray. Turn the flame down a little lower, cover, and let the chopped onions and garlic steam in their own juices. If you baste, use wine, tomato juice, lemon juice, or broth instead of fatty pan drippings. And by all means, avoid self-basting turkeys or chickens, which are always high in added fat.

Before you serve or thicken a sauce or soup, let the liquid cool. The fat will rise to the top and you can skim it off easily. Chill homemade or canned soups and broths and skim off the fat before you heat them up. You can also let pan drippings stand a few minutes before preparing your gravy. The fat will rise and you can pour it away, leaving the more flavorful juices. Thicken this remaining liquid with cornstarch mixed in water or with flour mixed in buttermilk to replace the standard flour/fat gravy base.

If you're preparing a dish that calls for sautéed ground meat, be sure to pour off all the fat after you've browned the meat. You don't need the fat for flavor if you're going to use the meat.

For sauces and gravies that call for sour cream or heavy cream, substitute plain low-fat yogurt. To prevent the yogurt from separating, mix one tablespoon of cornstarch with one tablespoon of yogurt and stir it into the remaining yogurt; add to the sauce or gravy. Heat over medium heat, just until thickened, and serve right away. When you make creamed soups or white sauces, use low-fat or skim milk rather than cream or whole milk. You can even try non-fat evaporated milk for these recipes. They come out thick and creamy, but have no fat.

Recipe Repair

Just because you're In Control, it doesn't mean you can't use your favorite recipes anymore. Often the ingredients can be modified to make an old standby lower in fat.

When a Recipe Calls For	Use Instead	This Lowers
1 tablespoon butter	¾ tablespoon oil	fat and cholesterol
1 cup solid fat (butter, margarine, lard, shortening)	⅔ cup oil	fat and cholesterol
butter	margarine	cholesterol
any fat	¼ less	fat
1 whole egg	2 egg whites	fat and cholesterol
1 cup whole milk	1 cup low-fat milk **or** skim milk	fat and cholesterol
1 cup sour cream	1 cup buttermilk **or** low-fat yogurt	fat and cholesterol
regular cheese	low-fat **or** part-skim cheese	fat
chocolate chips	raisins	fat
nuts	raisins **or** wheat bran	fat
sausage	ground turkey	fat
any meat	less meat, trimmed well	fat and cholesterol
duck or goose	chicken **or** turkey	fat
chicken or turkey, with skin	chicken **or** turkey, without skin	fat
fish canned in oil	fish canned in water	fat

More Kitchen Tips

Here are a few more cooking tips to reduce fat when you cook.

- Use cooking spray instead of greasing baking pans.
- Use whipped or diet margarine, whipped butter, and whipped or light cream cheese. But go easy with all of these anyway.
- Use butter sprinkles to top vegetables, pasta, rice, or potatoes, to get a buttery flavor without the fat.

- Make meat loaf, meatballs, and hamburgers with ground round or ground turkey instead of the fattier ground chuck. Try a mixture of the two when making meat loaf or meatballs. You'll be surprised to find that it tastes just like ground beef.
- Mix regular mayonnaise with nonfat plain yogurt in equal amounts for tuna, potato, and other salads.
- Top a baked potato with nonfat plain yogurt and chives instead of sour cream and chives.
- Mix your favorite salad dressing with nonfat plain yogurt or buttermilk for a creamy lower-fat version. (A handy buttermilk substitute for salad dressing or cooking is 1 cup of skim milk to which you add one tablespoon of vinegar; let sit for five to ten minutes at room temperature.)
- "Sauté" mushrooms in the microwave: Just slice or quarter them and put them in a microwave-proof cup or bowl, cover (but leave room for the steam to escape), and cook on medium-high for just a few minutes—with no fat at all. They'll exude a wonderful juice and can be added right away to sauces, soups, and entrées. (Remember the microwave rule: The minute you can smell the food cooking, you should check on it.)
- Don't add breadcrumbs to ground meat or poultry; they soak up the fat in the meat rather than let it drip off in the cooking. Try grated raw carrots or celery instead.
- Try leaving the butter or margarine off. A toasted bagel with jam or honey is every bit as good. Pancakes with syrup *and* butter? They taste just fine without the butter. Hot muffins don't need butter and neither does fresh bread; in fact, their own taste will come through better without it. Some cooks put butter or margarine on pasta after it has been cooked to keep it from sticking *before* it's drowned in sauce. Needless fat! If it gets sticky in the colander, refresh it by pouring boiling water over it again.
- Make croutons for soups and salads in the microwave without adding any fat, instead of sautéing them in butter.

See Super Start (beginning on page 55) and Getting Ahead (beginning on page 142) for even more ideas on cooking without added fat.

It Won't Be Long...

... before you master these techniques of low-fat cooking and come up with lots more of your own. Just remember that there are dozens of ways to add moisture without fat, and that when you remove hidden fat you almost never know the difference. Once you've learned to adapt your favorite meals you'll be amazed at how much fat you're attacking! And there's a very good chance you'll quickly come to prefer the lighter, lower-fat version, health benefits aside, based on nothing but pure taste.

Remember, when you're in the control center, you're In Control!

12 *In Control When You're Eating Out*

SELECTING LOW-FAT RESTAURANT FOOD

Picture this: You're in your favorite restaurant with good friends, celebrating a special birthday or anniversary. You open the menu and look at all the wonderful choices. Then you panic. *How* are you going to stay In Control here?

Take a deep breath . . . and look at the menu again. Then close your eyes and visualize the Fat Attack Target. Chances are there are more choices to pick from than you realized. Entrées with lots of pasta, rice, and beans are a good start. There's probably a basket of bread on the table already. A restaurant that doesn't serve some type of salad would be pretty unusual. Starting to feel better already? This isn't going to be such a bad night after all!

Always Remember

You are In Control, not the restaurant kitchen or the waiter. You can order and enjoy the meal you want. Restaurants are getting more and more used to feeding health-conscious people, so don't be shy about asking your waiter for skim milk instead of cream, margarine instead of butter, and salad dressing, sauce, and gravy on the side (so that you can control just how much you eat). If you're not sure how a dish is prepared, ask. You can always request that your choice be "dry broiled" or served "plain." These requests are easy and most restaurants are happy to accommodate. Remember, they want you to come back.

Now, if you've been In Control for over a month and you want to throw caution to the wind and eat whatever you'd like tonight—go ahead. Tomorrow you can balance tonight's choices by tracking your fat more carefully. Or when you know you're going out for a special meal such as tonight's, plan the earlier part of the day to be as fat free as possible.

Start Your Meal Light

A clear soup such as onion soup (minus the buttery toast and cheese), Manhattan clam chowder, or chicken broth with rice, noodles, or vegetables is a good starter. Other low-fat starters are oysters (raw, baked, or steamed), steamed mussels, steamed or raw clams (not baked with breadcrumbs and butter), and shrimp or crab cocktail.

And, of course, a salad. Ask for your dressing on the side, and stick with oil and vinegar if possible; that way you can use only the amount you want, and you can use more vinegar than oil. If you're dying for a creamy dressing, try this trick: Dip the tip of your fork in the dressing, then spear some salad. You'll get the taste you're after with far less fat.

New Options for Main Courses

There's more than one way to order a main course. If the main dish portions are large, order two appetizers instead, and ask that one be served as your main course. Diners are notorious for large portions, but most will let you split a meal between two people. Or don't be embarrassed to eat half and take the rest home. People do it all the time.

You can also request two salads. A large salad to munch on offers the satisfaction of chewing and reduces the temptation to eat higher-fat foods. Main dish salads are often loaded with cheese, eggs, and meat. Ask that yours be made with less, or take half the cheese and meat off the salad and request to take it home. Eat the egg whites but leave the yolks, and ask the waiter to hold the olives unless you really love them and have made room for them in your fat allowance that day.

If items that you have trouble resisting have a mysterious way of just appearing on your table, take a small amount and then make sure the waiter makes them disappear. You can always ask for a little more, like another pat or two of butter. It's better to do that than to make it all disappear yourself.

The Icing on the Cake

Desserts can be tough to resist. Splurge on special fruit like raspberries, without the cream. Or pick a fruit pie or tart and leave the crust—and the fat—behind. Sorbets and sherbets are good alternatives to high-fat ice cream and whipped cream desserts.

But you don't really have to be so virtuous all the time. You can pick your favorite and take half home. Share half with a friend, or just leave half behind. If you eat the whole dessert, enjoy it—but balance the extra fat you have tonight with less fat tomorrow.

You Can Go Anywhere

There's no restaurant that's "off limits" when you're In Control. Here are some great suggestions for choosing foods at a variety of different places:

Type	Order Often	Order Less Often
Chinese	Steamed dishes	Fried noodles
	Stir-fried dishes	Deep-fried dishes
	Plain rice	Fried rice
	Steamed dumplings	Fried dumplings
	Clear soups	Egg drop soup
	Steamed wontons	Fried wontons
	Fortune cookies	Egg rolls
	Fruit desserts	Spareribs
	Vegetable mixtures	Egg foo yong
	Lo mein dishes	Peking duck
	Bean curd	Dishes with nuts
French	Steamed shellfish	Butter sauces
	Grilled fresh fish	Blue cheese
	Squab	Cream sauce
	Broiled lean meat	Rich pastries
	Marengo sauce	Allemande sauce
	Diablo sauce	Béarnaise sauce
	Fresh fruit and cheese	Pâté
	French bread	
	Sorbet	
	Niçoise salad	
	Marrons glacés	
Italian	Plain pasta	Deep-fried dishes
	Pasta primavera (no cream)	Cream sauces
		Meat sauces
	Marinara sauce	Sausage
	Tomato-based sauce	Frittata
	Chicken	Cheesecake
	Fish	Custard pastries
	Red clam sauce	Garlic bread
	Cacciatore	Whipped-cream pastries
	Italian bread	Neapolitan ice cream
	Breadsticks	Salami
	Minestrone soup	
	Pasta e fagioli	
	Steamed artichokes	
	Italian ice	
	Fresh fruit	
	Fruit poached in wine	

Type	Order Often	Order Less Often
Mexican	Chicken enchiladas (without cheese)	Nachos
	Gazpacho	Fried tortilla chips
	Lean beef fajitas	Sour cream
	Chicken fajitas	Avocados
	Bean burritos (without cheese)	Guacamole
		Refried beans
	Salsa	Cheese sauce
	Steamed tortillas	
	Spanish rice	
	Rice and beans	
	Bean soup	
Indian	Chick-peas	Deep-fried dishes
	Mixed-bean salad	Fried flatbread
	Tandoori chicken or seafood	
	Cucumber with yogurt	
	Chutney	
	Baked flatbreads	
	Steamed breads	
	Yogurt	
	Kabobs	
	Rice	
	Dal	
	Sharbat	
Greek	Grape leaves	Lemon soup
	Roast lamb	Moussaka
	Kabobs	Pastitsio
	Grilled or roasted chicken	Baklava
	Bean soup	Cheese pie or pudding
	Lentil soup	Spinach pie
	Marinated seafood	Olives
	Pilaf	
	Grilled fish	
	Yogurt and cucumber	

American	Roast turkey	Fried chicken
	Roast chicken	Steak
	Broiled fish	Spareribs
	Baked potato	Buttered biscuits
	Plain vegetables	Creamy salad dressing
	Salad	Gravy
	Corn on the cob	Coleslaw
	Filet mignon	Prime ribs
	Sourdough bread	Fried fish
Fast Food	Plain hamburger	Double hamburger
	Salad-bar greens	Cheeseburger
	Salad-bar beans	French fries
	Salad-bar vegetables	Onion rings
	Salad-bar fruits	Fried chicken
	Baked potato	Fish fillet sandwich
	Plain pizza	Pepperoni pizza
	Corn on the cob	Gravy
	Mashed potatoes	Cheese sauce
	Roast beef sandwich	Shakes

Take a look at the left-hand column again. And you thought there was nothing you could eat?

13 *The Picture of Health*
HOW DO YOU LOOK?

What does good health mean to you? Where do *you* think it comes from? When you picture a healthy, energetic, "fit" person, do you picture yourself?

If you've been following the Fat Attack Plan—or even if you've just read all about it—you'd probably say that good health is largely a product of what you eat. And it certainly is. Following a low-fat eating plan is one of the best ways we know to maintain the weight that's right for you and to prevent a variety of serious illnesses.

That's why we created the Fat Attack Plan. It's why we believe in it and why we follow it. And it's why we hope you'll follow it, too. It can, quite literally, change your life! But there's more to living a healthy life than just eating right. And just as you control what you eat, so too can you control many of the other factors that contribute to good health.

Maybe you feel like the picture of health already. Or maybe you don't —but wouldn't you like to? To a large extent, *you* paint the picture. So why not step back for a moment and see what that picture really looks like?

Circle your answer to each of the following questions.

1. I eat two or more servings of vegetables each day. (*Examples:* ½ cup broccoli, ½ cup carrots, ½ cup zucchini, one tomato.)
   A Yes   B Sometimes   C Never

2. I eat one serving of a vitamin A–rich food each day. (*Examples:* carrots, spinach, squash, mango.)
   A Yes   B Sometimes   C Never

3. I eat two or more servings of fruit each day. (*Examples:* banana, mango, apple, grapes.)
   A Yes   B Sometimes   C Never

4. I eat one serving of vitamin C–rich food each day. (*Examples:* orange, grapefruit, tomato, or their juices; strawberries, cantaloupe, coleslaw.)
   A Yes   **B** Sometimes   **C** Never

5. I drink two glasses of low-fat milk each day, or I eat two servings of low-fat dairy foods each day. (*Examples:* cheese, yogurt.)
   A Yes   **B** Sometimes   **C** Never

6. I eat at least two servings of lean meat, fish, poultry, dried peas, or beans each day.
   A Yes   **B** Sometimes   **C** Never

7. I eat no more than three to four eggs each week.
   A Yes   **B** Sometimes   **C** Never

8. I eat four or more servings of bread, cereal, rice, noodles, or pasta each day.
   A Yes   **B** Sometimes   **C** Never

9. I eat whole-grain breads and cereals.
   A Yes   **B** Sometimes   **C** Never

10. I eat no more than one serving of cake, cookies, pastries, baked goods, or candy each day.
    A Yes   **B** Sometimes   **C** Never

11. I limit my use of salt and salty foods each day. (*Examples:* ham, bacon, snack chips, pickles, canned, or dry soup.)
    A Yes   **B** Sometimes   **C** Never

12. I limit my use of fats and oils each day. (*Examples:* butter, margarine, salad dressings, fried foods.)
    A Yes   **B** Sometimes   **C** Never

13. I eat breakfast.
    A Yes   **B** Sometimes   **C** Never

14. I eat when I'm hungry, not when the clock says it's mealtime.
    A Yes   **B** Sometimes   **C** Never

15. I snack.
    A Yes   **B** Sometimes   **C** Never

16. I drink no more than two alcoholic drinks each day. (*Examples:* beer, wine, cocktail.)
    A Yes   **B** Sometimes   **C** Never

17. Each day I walk a total of:
    A 5 miles or more   **B** 3 miles or more   **C** Less than a mile

18. Each day I climb a total of:

   A 10 or more   **B** 5 or more   **C** Less than 1
      staircases   staircases   staircase

19. Each week I exercise:

   A 30 minutes,   **B** 30 minutes, less **C** Not at all
      every other day   than three
                   times a week

20. I regularly practice other good health habits.

   A Yes   **B** Sometimes   **C** Never

How does your picture look? If you have ten or more A's, you're doing well. If not, just remember that as time goes on, you can always go back and test yourself again. And no matter what your score is, your goal is to have more A's than you had the previous time—and always to have as many A's as possible. You'll find that as you incorporate more sensible, low-fat eating habits and other healthy practices into your daily routine, the A's will pile up very quickly.

What You Eat

The chances are good that you have already embarked on a program of low-fat living and are making sensible food choices every day. You already know how much your diet has to do with your health, and that getting the excess fat out of your diet is the one thing you have to be concerned about if good health is what you're after.

If you've been following the Fat Attack Plan, you may now be at your ideal weight and keeping your fat consumption well "In Control." You're probably feeling and looking great—the picture of health!

But if your picture still needs a little touching up, that's fine, too. Just remember, every day you have a new chance to attack your fat! You have all the tools you need, and you know exactly what to do to keep your eating plan—and your health—on course. With the Fat Attack principles to guide you, you'll be In Control in no time.

Alcoholic Beverages

It's best to keep your alcoholic beverage intake moderate. What does that mean? In technical terms, no more than one ounce of pure alcohol per day. In practical terms, it means no more than two four-ounce glasses of wine, *or* two twelve-ounce beers (regular or light), *or* two jiggers of hard liquor, per day. While drinking too much alcohol can promote health problems, such as high blood pressure, cancer, digestive upset, and mineral imbalances, moderate intakes may even be beneficial—although no one is quite sure why.

Exercise

You probably already know that exercise and low-fat eating are a natural combination. In fact, many people would rank exercise as the next most important thing to diet when it comes to "being healthy." And it's no wonder. Both improve your health, and many exercisers truly prefer to follow a low-fat diet. The two just seem to go hand in hand.

Of course, you should check with your doctor before you begin any program of strenuous physical activity. But once you've found a program that's right for you, you'll no doubt find that exercise is enjoyable and makes you feel better. It has many distinct health benefits, too. For one thing, it helps reduce body fat. Exercise strengthens your cardiovascular system, increases muscle, strengthens your bones by increasing their calcium content, and even helps reduce stress. Moreover, exercise helps improve your ratio of "good" HDL cholesterol to "bad" LDL cholesterol.

A study done with graduates of Harvard University showed that alumni who used up two thousand calories a week in exercise lived longer. When their walking, climbing stairs, and playing sports totaled two thousand calories or more each week, there was a *28* percent lower death rate in these people than in those who were less active. While the Harvard alumni may not be typical of the general population, the results of this study certainly support the long-held belief that exercise is good for you.

Your body spends energy just by staying alive, but exercise, of course, burns up additional energy—which can help you maintain your target weight. Yes, it's true that you'd have to walk five city blocks to use up the fat calories in one pat of butter, but *if you're active,* the amount of energy you use up during the course of the day can add up. That's why it's important to do things like walking instead of riding, and climbing stairs instead of taking an elevator—whenever you can. Using up that little extra bit of energy many times each day will help you maintain your weight *and* your good health.

Picture Yourself

Healthy, fit, feeling and looking wonderful—isn't this the way you'd like to be? You can! A longer, healthier life is a real possibility when you take good care of yourself. In addition to eating well, exercising, and watching how much you drink, it's important to have regular physical examinations, to try not to smoke, and to reduce stress as much as possible.

Having a social support network is also critical, as is protecting yourself against accidents and simply getting enough sleep.

But what better place to start taking good care of yourself than with what you eat every day? Build your meals around nutritious, low-fat foods. Choose your fat foods carefully. Track your fat. Eat in moderation. When you do all these things, you'll be painting yourself into the picture of health. So go ahead. Attack your fat! Give yourself the advantage of good food *and* good health—every day of your life!

Bibliography

Acheson, K. J.; Flatt, J. P.; and Jequrer, E. "Glycogen Synthesis versus Lipogenesis After 500 g Carbohydrate Meal in Man." *Metabolism* 31 (1982): 1234.

Albanes, D. "Total Calories, Body Weight and Tumor Incidence in Mice." *Cancer Research* 47 (1987): 8.

Allison, F. G. "Fats and Insulin," Letter in *Canadian Medical Association Journal* 141 (1989): 13.

American Cancer Society. "Nutrition and Cancer: Cause and Prevention." *American Cancer Society Special Report.* 1984.

American Diabetes Association, Inc. and American Dietetic Association. "Exchange Lists for Meal Planning." 1986.

American Heart Association. "Dietary Guidelines for Healthy American Adults: A statement for Physicians and Health Professionals by the Nutrition Committee." 1986.

American Heart Association. *Dietary Treatment of Hypercholesterolemia: A Handbook for Counselors.* 1988.

American Institute for Cancer Research. *Get Fit, Trim Down.* Information Series, Part III. 1989.

Anderson, K. M.; Castelli, W. P.; and Levy, D. "Cholesterol and Mortality: 30 Years of Follow-up from the Framingham Study." *Journal of the American Medical Association* 257 (1987): 2176.

Arky, R.; Wylie-Rosett, J.; and El-Beheri, B. "Examination of Current Dietary Recommendations of Individuals with Diabetes Mellitus." *Diabetes Care* 5 (1982): 59.

Bezwoda, W. R.; Torrance, J. D.; Bothwell, T. H.; Macphail, A. P.; Graham, B.; and Mills, W. "Iron Absorption from Red and White Wines." *Scandinavian Journal of Haematology* 34 (1985): 121.

Bonanome, A., and Grundy, S. M. "Effect of Dietary Stearic Acid on Plasma Cholesterol and Lipoprotein Levels." *New England Journal of Medicine* 318 (1988): 1244.

Bray, George A. "Obesity: Definition, Diagnosis, Disadvantages." *Medical Journal of Australia* 142 (1985): 82.

Camargo, C. A., Jr.; Williams, P. T.; Vranizan, K. M.; Albers, J. J.; and Wood, P. D. "The Effect of Moderate Alcohol Intake on Serum Apolipoproteins A-I and A-II." *Journal of the American Medical Association* 253 (1985): 2854.

Carroll, M. D.; Abraham, S. A.; and Dresser, C. M.; "Dietary Intake Source Data: US, 1976–80 (HANES II)." *Vital and Health Statistics,* Series 11, no. 231 (1983), DHHS-Pub. No. (PHS) 83-1681.

Carroll, M. D.; Abraham, S. A.; Dresser, C. M.; and Johnson, C. L. "Dietary Intake Source Data: US, 1971–74 (HANES I)." *Vital and Health Statistics,* Series 11 (1979), PHS79-1221.

Cassidy, M. M.; Lightfood, F. G.; Grau, L. E.: Story, J. A.; Kritchevsky, D.; and Vahouny, G. V. "Effect of Chronic Intake of Dietary Fibers on the Ultrastructural Topography of Rat Jejunum and Colon: A Scanning Electron Microscopy Study." *American Journal of Clinical Nutrition* 34 (1981): 218.

Chandra, R. K. "Nutrition, Immunity, and Infection: Present Knowledge and Future Directions." *Lancet* (1983): 688.

Chandra, R. K. "Nutritional Regulation of Immunity and Infection: From Epidemiology to Phenomenology to Clinical Practice." *Journal of Pediatric Gastroenterology* 5 (1986): 844.

Committee on Diet and Health, Food and Nutrition Board, Commission on Life Sciences, National Research Council. *Diet and Health, Implications for Reducing Chronic Disease, Executive Summary.* Washington, DC: National Academy Press, 1989.

Consensus Development Panel, National Institutes of Health. "Treatment of Hypertryglyceridemia." *Journal of the American Medical Association* 251 (1984): 1196.

Council on Scientific Affairs. "Dietary Fiber and Health." *Journal of the American Medical Association* 262 (1989): 542.

Danforth, E. "Diet and Obesity." *American Journal of Clinical Nutrition* 41 (1985): 1132.

Diamond, E. L. "The Role of Anger and Hostility in Essential Hypertension and Coronary Heart Disease." *Psychological Bulletin* 92 (1982): 410.

DiLorenzo, C.; Williams, C. M.: Hajnal, F.; and Valenzuela, J. E. "Pectin Delays Gastric Emptying and Increases Satiety in Obese Subjects." *Gastroenterology* 95 (1988): 1211.

Drewnowski, A. "Obesity and Taste: New Approaches." *Current Concepts and Perspectives in Nutrition.* Nutrition Information Center 8 (1984): 1.

Drewnowski, A., and Greenwood, M.C.R. "Cream and Sugar, Human Preferences for High Fat Food." *Physiology and Behavior* 30 (1983): 629.

Droen, D. M.; Frey-Hewitt, B.; Ellsworth, N.; Williams, P. T.; Terry, R. B.; and Wood, P. D. "Dietary Fat: Carbohydrate Ratio and Obesity in Middle-aged Men." *American Journal of Clinical Nutrition* 47 (1988): 995.

Ernst, N. D.; Cleeman, J.; Mullis, R.; Sooter-Bochenek, J.; and Van Horn, L. "The National Cholesterol Education Program: Implications for Dietetic Practitioners from the Adult Treatment Panel Recommendations." *Journal of the American Dietetic Association* 88 (1988): 1401.

"Evaluation of the Health Aspects of Pectin and Pectinates as Food Ingredients." FASEB/SCOGS Report 81 (NTIS PB 274–477) 1977.

Flatt, J. P. "Dietary Fat, Carbohydrate Balance and Weight Maintenance: Effect of Exercise." *American Journal of Clinical Nutrition* 45 (1987): 296.

Freiherr, G. "Pattern of Body Fat May Predict Occurrence of Diabetes." *Research Resources Reporter* USDA VI (1982): 1.

Freydberg, N., and Gortner, W. A. *The Food Additives Book.* Mt. Vernon, N.Y.: Consumers Union, 1982.

Goldman, P. "Coffee and Health: What's Brewing?" *New England Journal of Medicine* 310 (1984): 783.

Greenberg, L. A. "Alcohol and Emotional Behavior." In *Alcohol and Civilization,* S. P. Lucia (ed.), 1963.

Human Nutrition Information Service, USDA. "Nationwide Food Consumption Survey, Continuing Survey of Food Intakes by Individuals, Women 19–50 Years and Their Children 1–5 Years, 4 Days, 1985." NFCS, CSF11, Pub. No. 85-4, 1987.

Institute of Food Technologists' Expert Panel on Food Safety & Nutrition. "Low-calorie Foods, a Scientific Status Summary." *Food Technology* 43 (1989): 432

Jenkins, D. J. A.; Wolever, T.; Vuksan, V.; Brighenti, F.; Cunnane, S. C.; Venketeshwer, R.; Jenkins, A. L.; Buckley, G.; Patten, R.; Singer, W.; Corey, P.; and Josse, R. G. "Nibbling versus Gorging: Metabolic Advantages of Increased Meal Frequency." *New England Journal of Medicine* 321 (1989): 929.

Katch, F. I., and McArdle, W. D. *Nutrition, Weight Control, and Exercise.* Boston: Houghton Mifflin Company, 1983.

Kinosian, B. P., and Eisenberg, J. M. "Cutting into Cholesterol." *Journal of the American Medical Association* 259 (1988): 2249.

Kris-Etherton, K.; Krummel, D.; Russell, M. E.; Dreon, D.; Mackey, S.; Borchers, J.; and Wood, P. D. "The Effect of Diet on Plasma Lipids, Lipoproteins, and Coronary Heart Disease, National Cholesterol Education Program." *Journal of the American Dietetic Association* 88 (1988): 1373.

Kune, S. "Case-control Study of Dietary Etiological Factors: The Melbourne Colorectal Cancer Study." *Nutrition & Cancer,* 9 (1987): 21.

LaCroix, A. Z.; Mead, L. A.; Liang, K-Y.; Thomas, C. B.; and Pearson, T. A. "Coffee Consumption and the Incidence of Coronary Heart Disease." *New England Journal of Medicine* 315 (1986): 977.

Lane, H. W., and Carpenter, J. T. "Breast Cancer: Incidence, Nutritional Concerns, and Treatment Approaches." *Journal of the American Dietetic Association* 87 (1987): 765.

Langford, H. G.; Blaufox, M. D.; Oberman, A.; Hawkins, M.: Curb, J. D.; Cutter, G. R.; Wassertheil-Smoker, W.; Pressel, S.; Babcock, C.; Abernethy, J. D.; Hotchkiss, J.; and Tyler, M. "Dietary Therapy Slows the Return of Hypertension After Stopping Prolonged Medication." *Journal of the American Medical Association* 253 (1985): 657.

Lanza, E., and Butrum, R. R. "A Critical Review of Food Fiber Analysis and Data." *Journal of the American Dietetic Association* 86 (1986): 732.

Leonard, T. K. "The Effect of Caffeine on Various Body Systems." *Journal of the American Dietetic Association* 87 (1987): 1048.

Lopes, E. da C. da F. "The Relation Between Cancer of the Colon and Rectum and Nutrition in Rio de Janeiro." *Archivos Latinoamericanos de Nutricion* 36 (1986): 282.

McCarron, D. A. "Is Calcium More Important Than Sodium in the Pathogenesis of Essential Hypertension?" *Hypertension* 7 (1985): 607.

McCarron, D. A. and Morris, C. D. "Blood Pressure Response to Oral Calcium in Persons with Mild to Moderate Hypertension." *Annals of Internal Medicine* 103 (1985): 825.

McGill, P. E. "Gouty Arthritis in the Geriatric Patient." *Geriatric Medicine Today* 6 (1987): 59.

Maclure, K. M.; Hayes, K. C.; Colditz, G. A.; Stampfer, M. J.; Speizer, F. E.; and Willett, W. C. "Weight, Diet, and the Risk of Symptomatic Gallstones in Middle-aged Women." *New England Journal of Medicine* 321 (1989): 563.

Manson, J. E. "Body Weight and Longevity: A Reassessment." *Journal of the American Medical Association* 257 (1987): 353.

Mellin, L. *Shapedown.* San Francisco: Balboa Publishing, 1983.

National Cancer Institute. "Cancer Prevention." NIH Pub. No. 84-2671, 1984.

National Cholesterol Education Program, National Heart, Lung, Blood Institute. "So You Have High Blood Cholesterol." NIH Pub. No. 87-2922, 1987.

National Cholesterol Education Program. Report of the Expert Panel on Detection, Evaluation, and Treatment of High Blood Cholesterol in Adults. NIH Pub. No. 89-2925, 1989.

National Institutes of Health. "Health Implications of Obesity Consensus Development Conference Statement." *Annals of Internal Medicine* 103 (1985): 1073.

"New Findings on Palm Oil." *Nutrition Reviews* 45 (1987): 205

"Nutrition Update: Fat/Cholesterol." *Dairy Council Digest* 55 (1984): 1.

Ockene, I. S., and Ockene, J. K. "Coffee Consumption and the Incidence of Coronary Heart Disease." Letter in *New England Journal of Medicine* 316 (1987): 945

O'Connor, T. P. "Dietary Fat, Calories and Cancer." *Contemporary Nutrition* 10 (1985): 1.

Paffenbarger, R. S.; Hyde, R. T.; Alvin, L. W.; and Hsieh, C-C. "Physical Activity, All-cause Mortality, and Longevity of College Alumni." *New England Journal of Medicine* 314 (1986): 605.

Patterson, B. H. "Food Choices and the Cancer Guidelines." *American Journal of Public Health* 78 (1988): 282.

Public Health Service HHS. "The Surgeon General's Report on Nutrition and Health." DHHS (PHS) Pub. No. 88-50210, 1988.

Raymond, C. A. "Biology, Culture, Dietary Changes Conspire to Increase Incidence of Obesity." *Journal of the American Medical Association* 256 (1986): 2157.

Romieu, I.; Willet, W. C.; Stampfer, M. J.; Colditz, A.; Sampson, L.; Rosner, B.; Hennekens, C. H.; Speizer, F. E. "Energy Intake and other Determinants of Relative Weight." *American Journal Clinical Nutrition* 47 (1988): 406.

Ryttig, K. R.; Tellnes, G.; Haegh, L. H.; Boe, E.; and Fagerthun, H. "A Dietary Fibre Supplement and Weight Maintenance After Weight Reduction: A Randomized, Double-blind, Placebo-controlled Long-term Trial." *International Journal of Obesity* 13 (1988): 165.

Sandhu, K. S.; El Samahi, M. M.; Mena, I; Dooley, C. P.; and Valenzuela, J. E. "Effect of Pectin on Gastric Emptying and Gastroduodenal Motility in Normal Subjects." *Gastroenterology* 92 (1987): 486.

Simopoulos, A. P. and Van Itallie, T. B. "Body Weight, Health, and Longevity." *Annals of Internal Medicine* 100 (1985): 285.

Spiller, G. A.; Chernoff, M. C.; Hill, R. A.; Gates, J. E.; Nassar, J. J.; and Shipley, E. A. "Effect of Purified Cellulose, Pectin, and a Low-residue Diet on Fecal Volatile Fatty Acids, Transit Time, and Fecal Weight in Humans." *American Journal of Clinical Nutrition* 33 (1980): 754.

Thorpe, C. J., and Caprinio, J. A. "Gall Bladder Disease: Current Trends and Treatments." *American Journal of Nursing* 80 (1980): 2181.

Threbaud, D. "Energy Cost of Glucose Storage in Human Subjects During Glucose-insulin Infusions." *American Journal of Physiology* 244 (1983): E216.

Toniolo, P.; Riboli, E.; Protta, F.; Charrel, M.; and Cappa, A.P.M. "Calorie-providing Nutrients and Risk of Breast Cancer." *Journal of the National Cancer Institute* 81 (1989): 278.

US–Japan Cooperative Cancer Research Program Conference. "Causative and Modifying Factors in Digestive Tract Cancer." *Cancer Research* 47 (1987): 922.

Van Itallie, T. B. "Health Implications of Overweight and Obesity in the United States." *Annals of Internal Medicine* 103 (1985): 9.

"Weight Control." *Dairy Council Digest* 55 (1984): 1.

Wheeler, M. L.; Delahanty, L.; and Wylie-Rosett, J. "Diet and Exercise in Noninsulin-dependent Diabetes Mellitus: Implications for Dietitians from the NIH Consensus Development Conference." *Journal of the American Dietetic Association* 87 (1987): 480.

Willett, W. C. "Diet and Cancer—An Overview," Part I. *New England Journal of Medicine* 310 (1984): 633.

Willett, W. C. "Diet and Cancer—An Overview," Part II. *New England Journal of Medicine* 310 (1984): 697.

Williams, P. T.; Wood, P. D.; Vranizan, K. M.; Albers, J. J.; Garay, S. C.; and Taylor, C. B. "Coffee Intake and Elevated Apolipoprotein b Levels in Men." *Journal of the American Medical Association* 253 (1985): 1407.

Wine Institute. *Wine and Medical Practice.* San Francisco, 1979.

Wynder, E. "Dietary Fat and Fiber and Colon Cancer." *Seminars in Oncology* X (1983): 264.

Yetiv, J. Z. "Clinical Applications of Fish Oils." *Journal of the American Medical Association* 260 (1988): 665.